Buprenorphine Therapy
of Opiate Addiction

FORENSIC SCIENCE AND MEDICINE

Steven B. Karch, MD, SERIES EDITOR

BUPRENORPHINE THERAPY OF OPIATE ADDICTION, edited by **Pascal Kintz** and **Pierre Marquet**, 2002

ON-SITE DRUG TESTING, edited by **Amanda J. Jenkins** and **Bruce A. Goldberger**, 2002

BENZODIAZEPINES AND GHB: DETECTION AND PHARMACOLOGY, edited by **Salvatore J. Salamone**, 2002

TOXICOLOGY AND CLINICAL PHARMACOLOGY OF HERBAL PRODUCTS, edited by **Melanie Johns Cupp**, 2000

CRIMINAL POISONING: INVESTIGATIONAL GUIDE FOR LAW ENFORCEMENT, TOXICOLOGISTS, FORENSIC SCIENTISTS, AND ATTORNEYS, by **John H. Trestrail, III**, 2000

A PHYSICIAN'S GUIDE TO CLINICAL FORENSIC MEDICINE, edited by **Margaret M. Stark**, 2000

BRAIN IMAGING IN SUBSTANCE ABUSE: RESEARCH, CLINICAL, AND FORENSIC APPLICATIONS, edited by **Marc J. Kaufman**, 2000

BUPRENORPHINE THERAPY OF OPIATE ADDICTION

Edited by

Pascal Kintz, PharmD, PhD
Institute of Legal Medicine, Strasbourg, France
President, Societé Française de Toxicologie Analytique

Pierre Marquet, MD, PhD
Department of Pharmacology and Toxicology, University Hospital;
Professor of Pharmacology, Faculty of Medicine, Limoges University, Limoges, France

Foreword by

Albert D. Fraser
Clinical and Forensic Toxicologist, Queen Elizabeth II Health Sciences Centre and Professor of Pathology and Pharmacy, Dalhousie University, Halifax, Nova Scotia, Canada; President, International Association for Therapeutic Drug Monitoring and Clinical Toxicology, 2001–2003

Humana Press ※ Totowa, New Jersey

© 2002 Humana Press Inc.
999 Riverview Drive, Suite 208
Totowa, New Jersey 07512

www.humanapress.com

All rights reserved. No part of this book may be reproduced, stored in a retrieval system, or transmitted in any form or by any means, electronic, mechanical, photocopying, microfilming, recording, or otherwise without written permission from the Publisher.

The content and opinions expressed in this book are the sole work of the authors and editors, who have warranted due diligence in the creation and issuance of their work. The publisher, editors, and authors are not responsible for errors or omissions or for any consequences arising from the information or opinions presented in this book and make no warranty, express or implied, with respect to its contents.

This publication is printed on acid-free paper. ∞

ANSI Z39.48-1984 (American Standards Institute) Permanence of Paper for Printed Library Materials.

Cover design by Patricia F. Cleary.

For additional copies, pricing for bulk purchases, and/or information about other Humana titles, contact Humana at the above address or at any of the following numbers: Tel: 973-256-1699; Fax: 973-256-8341; E-mail: humana@humanapr.com, or visit our Website at www.humanapress.com

Photocopy Authorization Policy:

Authorization to photocopy items for internal or personal use, or the internal or personal use of specific clients, is granted by Humana Press Inc., provided that the base fee of US $10.00 per copy, plus US $00.25 per page, is paid directly to the Copyright Clearance Center at 222 Rosewood Drive, Danvers, MA 01923. For those organizations that have been granted a photocopy license from the CCC, a separate system of payment has been arranged and is acceptable to Humana Press Inc. The fee code for users of the Transactional Reporting Service is: [1-58829-031-X/02 $10.00 + $00.25].

Printed in the United States of America. 10 9 8 7 6 5 4 3 2 1

Library of Congress Cataloging in Publication Data

Buprenorphine therapy of opiate addiction / edited by Pascal Kintz, Pierre Marquet; foreword by Alan D. Fraser.
  p. ; cm.
  Includes bibliographical references and index.
  ISBN 1-58829-031-X (alk. paper)
  1. Opioid habit--Chemotherapy. 2. Buprenorphine. I. Kintz, Pascal. II. Marquet, Pierre.
  [DNLM: 1. Buprenorphine--pharmacology. 2. Buprenorphine--therapeutic use. 3. Opioid-Related Disorders--drug therapy. QV 92 B9447 2002]
  RC568.O45 B87 2002
  616.86'32061--dc21

2001039718

Foreword

It is a great pleasure to write a foreword to this new book on buprenorphine treatment in opiate dependency. Abuse of heroin is a major public health problem worldwide. In the United States alone, there are almost one million long-term users of heroin. Clinical- and laboratory-based investigators in many centers in France have written the largest number of chapters in this book. This is because French physicians and scientists have the most experience with high-dose buprenorphine treatment in opiate dependency. The experience and contributions of the French in both clinical- and laboratory-based studies provide a wealth of knowledge for other opiate treatment centers having less experience using buprenorphine. When one speaks about opiate dependency, one is primarily referring to heroin addiction, although addiction to many other opioids is a problem in various parts of the world. The first chapter discusses the important fundamental question whether substituting heroin for a surrogate opioid (such as methadone or buprenorphine) is a therapeutic treatment or meant to serve another purpose in society. In another chapter, long-term maintenance of opiate-dependent patients with high-dose buprenorphine is compared to methadone use. This is important information because of the significant differences between methadone and high-dose buprenorphine as maintenance therapies. There are major differences in the frequency of administration and delivery of buprenorphine compared to methadone today. Two chapters present how buprenorphine is currently prescribed and monitored in France and Australia.

Administration and monitoring of buprenorphine presents a great challenge in specific populations. Two chapters in this book describe the use of buprenorphine in the pregnant addict. The clinical and/or forensic laboratory plays an integral role in the assessment and monitoring of opiate-addicted patients since methadone was introduced clinically almost 40 years ago. The latest advances in analytical techniques for the determination of buprenorphine and metabolites in biological fluids and tissues are presented in another chapter. Analytical methods developed in toxicology laboratories and the interpretation of results are essential components of successful opiate addiction treatment programs. Diversion of surrogate opioids such as buprenorphine and the possibility of overdose/poisoning are always a concern. A chapter on buprenorphine poisoning is an important feature of *Buprenorpine Therapy of Opiate Addiction.*

A reference text on high-dose buprenorphine in the treatment of opioid addiction must cover all the key topics that treatment personnel and laboratory scientists in this field experience in their working environment. The broad scope and depth of topics covered by internationally known scientist and physician authors will make this book a valuable reference text for individuals working in the addiction field worldwide for many years.

Albert D. Fraser
Halifax, Nova Scotia
Canada

Preface

Buprenorphine is a semisynthetic opioid derivative, closely related to morphine and obtained from thebaine after a seven-step chemical procedure. At low doses, buprenorphine is a powerful analgesic, 25–40 times more potent than morphine, with mixed agonist/antagonist activity on opioid receptors. The drug is a partial μ receptor agonist and a κ receptor antagonist. It shows very slow dissociation from opiate receptors, which is one of the reasons for its long duration of action.

Buprenorphine is characterized by a weak oral bioavailability and, owing to its high lipid solubility, by low therapeutic concentrations.

Under the tradename Temgesic® at dosages of 0.2 mg, buprenorphine has been widely prescribed for about 20 years for the treatment of moderate to severe pain as well as in anesthesiology for premedication and/or anesthetic induction.

More recently, it also has been recognized as a medication of interest for the substitutive management of opiate-dependent individuals. Under the tradename Subutex®, a high-dosage formulation (0.4-, 2-, and 8-mg tablets for sublingual use) has been available in France since February 1996 in this specific indication. Today, this drug is largely used in France for the treatment of about 70,000 heroin addicts but can also be easily found on the black market.

The fatality risks incurred by the misuse of buprenorphine seem to arise through a combination of two practices: (1) association with other psychotropics, especially benzodiazepines and neuroleptics, and (2) improper use of the tablet form for intravenous administration or massive oral doses.

Special thanks must go to all the authors who accepted our request to write a chapter of what, we hope, is a worthwhile contribution to the literature. It was our intention to cover both theoretical and practical aspects of buprenorphine therapy in order to provide a reference book. As will be seen by the readers, pharmacology, controlled studies, clinical observations and experience, drug delivery, analytical challenges and postmortem forensic toxicology were reviewed by the different authors. We believe these chapters will provide readers not only with a comprehensive and well-documented survey of what other investigators have reported, but also with each author's critical evaluation of current knowledge in each of the areas surveyed.

Pascal Kintz, PharmD, PhD
Pierre Marquet, MD, PhD

Contents

Foreword by *Albert D. Fraser* v
Preface vii
Contributors xv

CHAPTER 1
Pharmacology of High-Dose Buprenorphine
Pierre Marquet 1
   1. Introduction 1
   2. Pharmacokinetic Properties 1
      2.1. Absorption and Bioavailability 1
      2.2. Distribution 3
      2.3. Metabolism 5
      2.4. Excretion 5
   3. Pharmacodynamic Properties 5
   4. Administration Schedules 8
   5. Clinical Effects of Buprenorphine 8
   6. Conclusion 9
   References 9

CHAPTER 2
Controlled Drug Administration Studies
of High-Dose Buprenorphine in Humans
Marilyn A. Huestis 13
   1. Introduction 13
   2. Bioavailability 14
   3. Dose-Effect Profiles 16
   4. Abuse Liability 16
   5. Toxicity 19
   6. Safety and Abuse Liability of High-Dose Intravenous Buprenorphine 21
   7. Conclusion 23
   References 24

Chapter 3

High-Dose Buprenorphine for Treatment of Opioid Dependence

Eric C. Strain **29**

1. Introduction 29
2. Buprenorphine Solution vs Tablets 30
3. Efficacy of Buprenorphine vs Placebo: *Clinical Trials* 31
   3.1. Summary of Placebo-Controlled Studies 34
4. Efficacy of Buprenorphine vs Other Medications:
   Clinical Trials 34
   4.1. Summary of Studies Comparing Buprenorphine
   to Other Medications 44
5. Safety and Side Effects of Buprenorphine 44
6. Summary and Conclusions 45
Acknowledgment 47
References 47

Chapter 4

Foreseeable Advantages and Limits of Buprenorphine-Naloxone Association

Michel Mallaret, Maurice Dematteis, Celine Villier,
Claude Elisabeth Barjhoux, and Chantal Gatignol **51**

1. Introduction 51
2. Advantages of Buprenorphine-Naloxone Association 52
   2.1. Advantages of Opiate-Naloxone Association: *Lessons of the Past* 52
      2.1.1. Epidemic of Pentazocine and Tripelennamine Abuse
      in the United States 52
      2.1.2. Epidemic of Analgesic Buprenorphine Abuse in New Zealand ... 53
   2.2. Buprenorphine and Naloxone:
   A Complex and Controversial Pharmacology 53
   2.3. Clinical Aspects 54
      2.3.1. Pharmacokinetic/Pharmacodynamic Advantages
      of Associated Naloxone in BupNx Combination 54
      2.3.2. Sublingual Naloxone in BupNx Tablets Does Not Decrease
      Buprenorphine Effects 55
      2.3.3. Sublingual Naloxone in BupNx Tablets Does Not Decrease
      Blockade Effects of Buprenorphine
      in Opioid-Dependent Patients 55
      2.3.4. Sublingual Naloxone in BupNx Tablets Does Not Precipitate
      Withdrawal Symptoms in Opioid-Dependent Patients 56
      2.3.5. Is the BupNx Combination Effective for Detoxification
      or Treatment of Depressive Symptoms
      in Opioid-Dependent Patients? 56

2.3.6. What Is the Abuse Liability of Intravenous BupNx Combination
　　　　　in Nonopioid-Dependent and Opioid-Dependent Patients?.......... 56
　　　2.3.7. Intravenous Naloxone May Decrease Respiratory Depression
　　　　　by Buprenorphine 58
　　　2.3.8. What Will Be the Epidemiological Consequences and Potential
　　　　　Economic Impact of the Use of BupNx Combination? 59
3. Limits of Buprenorphine-Naloxone Association 59
　3.1. Potential Risk of Inefficacy of Naloxone in BupNx Combination 59
　3.2. Abuse Liability of Intravenous BupNx Combination:
　　　Low But Still Possible 60
　3.3. Adverse Buprenorphine Reactions and Sublingual BupNx Combination ... 60
　　　3.3.1. Respiratory Depression 61
　　　3.3.2. Involuntary Overdoses 62
　　　3.3.3. Experimental Buprenorphine Hepatotoxicity 62
　3.4. Specific Risks in Office-Based Treatment (BupNx Combination)
　　　of Opiate Dependence 63
4. Conclusion 63
References 64

CHAPTER 5

Buprenorphine Maintenance Treatment in Primary Care:
*An Overview of the French Experience
and Insight Into the Prison Setting*

Marc Deveaux and Jean Vignau 69

1. Introduction 69
2. Implementation of BMT Through French Primary Care System 70
　2.1. A Late But Considerable Concession to Harm Reduction Paradigm 70
　2.2. Legal Framework of Therapeutic Use of Buprenorphine 70
　　　2.2.1. Essential Landmarks of French Health Services 70
　　　2.2.2. Opioid Maintenance Treatments 71
3. Observable Effects of French Policy 72
　3.1. Is BMT Accessible and Acceptable? 72
　3.2. Is BMT Safe? 72
　　　3.2.1. Data from Preregistration Studies 73
　　　3.2.2. Data from French Experience 74
　3.3. Is BMT Effective in Controlling Opiate Addiction and Preventing
　　　Subsequent Relapses? 75
4. Prison 76
　4.1. Drug Addicts in French Prisons 76
　4.2. Legal Framework of BMT in Prison 76
　4.3. Procedures in Loos-lez-Lille Prison 77
5. Conclusion 78
Acknowledgments 79
References 79

Chapter 6
Buprenorphine as a Viable Pharmacotherapy in Australia
John H. Lewis 83
1. Introduction 83
2. Buprenorphine 84
3. National Evaluation of Pharmacotherapies for Opioid Dependence 86
4. Conclusion 86
Acknowledgments 87
References 87

Chapter 7
Separative Techniques for Determination of Buprenorphine
Vincent Cirimele 89
1. Introduction 89
2. Determination of Buprenorphine in Blood 90
3. Determination of Buprenorphine in Urine 96
4. Determination of Buprenorphine in Biological Tissues 99
5. Determination of Buprenorphine in Hair 99
6. Conclusion 106
References 106

Chapter 8
Buprenorphine-Related Deaths
Pascal Kintz 109
1. Introduction 109
2. Forensic Aspects 110
3. Buprenorphine Fatalities 110
4. Conclusion 115
References 116

Chapter 9
Pharmacology of Opiates During Pregnancy and in Neonates
Pierre Marquet 119
1. Introduction 119
2. Perinatal Pharmacokinetics of Opiates 119
   2.1. *In Utero* 119
      2.1.1. Transfer Through Placenta and Distribution in Fetus 119
      2.1.2. Transfer Through Blood-Brain Barrier 120
   2.2. Postnatal 120

Contents   xiii

    3. Perinatal Pharmacodynamics of Opiates 120
        3.1. Opioid Receptors and Development of Embryos 120
        3.2. Perinatal Effects of Exogenous Opiates.. 121
            3.2.1. On Development 121
            3.2.2. On Opioid System 122
    4. Maintenance Treatments During Pregnancy 122
    References 123

CHAPTER 10

Case Study of Neonates Born to Mothers
   Undergoing Buprenorphine Maintenance Treatment
   *Pierre Marquet, Pierre Lavignasse, Jean-Michel Gaulier,
   and Gérard Lachâtre* *125*

    1. Introduction 125
    2. Clinical Findings 126
        2.1. Neonates Included 126
        2.2. Questionnaire and Toxicological Survey of Mothers 126
        2.3. Neonates' Outcomes 130
    3. Toxicological Investigations 130
        3.1. Materials and Methods 130
        3.2. Results 131
    4. Discussion 133
    5. Conclusion 134
    Acknowledgments 135
    References 135

CHAPTER 11

Buprenorphine and Pregnancy:
   *A Comparative, Multicenter Clinical Study
   of High-Dose Buprenorphine vs Methadone Maintenance*
   *Claude Lejeune, Sandrine Aubisson, Laurence Simmat-Durand,
   Fabrice Cneude, and Martine Piquet* *137*

    1. Introduction 137
    2. Materials and Methods 138
    3. Results 139
    4. Discussion 143
    5. Conclusion 145
    Acknowledgments 145
    References 145

Index *147*

Contributors

SANDRINE AUBISSON • Département des Sciences Sociales, La Sorbonne, Paris, France
CLAUDE ELISABETH BARJHOUX • CEIP, Pharmacology, University Hospital Grenoble, Grenoble, France
VINCENT CIRIMELE • Institute of Legal Medicine, Strasbourg, France
FABRICE CNEUDE • Neonatal Unit, Hospital Saint Antoine, Lille, France
MAURICE DEMATTEIS • CEIP, Pharmacology, University Hospital Grenoble, Grenoble, France
MARC DEVEAUX • Institute of Legal Medicine; Department of Pharmacy, University Hospital, Lille, France
ALBERT D. FRASER • Department of Pharmacy, Queen Elizabeth II Health Sciences Centre, Dalhousie University, Halifax, Nova Scotia, Canada
CHANTAL GATIGNOL • CEIP, Pharmacology, University Hospital Grenoble, Grenoble, France
JEAN-MICHEL GAULIER • Department of Pharmacology and Toxicology, University Hospital, Limoges, France
MARILYN A. HUESTIS • Intramural Research Program, National Institute on Drug Abuse, Baltimore, MD
PASCAL KINTZ • Institute of Legal Medicine, Strasbourg, France; President, Societé Française de Toxicologie Analytique
GÉRARD LACHÂTRE • Department of Pharmacology and Toxicology, University Hospital, Limoges, France
PIERRE LAVIGNASSE • Department of Pharmacology, University Hospital, Limoges, France
CLAUDE LEJEUNE • Groupe d'Etudes Grossesse et Addictions, Service de Néonatologie, Hôpital Louis Mourier, Colombes, France
JOHN H. LEWIS • Toxicology Unit, Pacific Laboratory Medicine Services, Northern Sydney Health, North Ryde, NSW, Australia
MICHEL MALLARET • CEIP, Pharmacology, University Hospital Grenoble, Grenoble, France

PIERRE MARQUET • Department of Pharmacology and Toxicology, University Hospital, Limoges, France
MARTINE PIQUET • Protection Maternelle et Infantile, Paris, France
LAURENCE SIMMAT-DURAND • Département des Sciences Sociales, La Sorbonne, Paris, France
ERIC C. STRAIN • Department of Psychiatry and Behavioral Sciences, Johns Hopkins University School of Medicine, Baltimore, MD
JEAN VIGNAU • Service d'Addictologie, Clinique de la Charité, University Hospital, Lille, France
CELINE VILLIER • CEIP, Pharmacology, University Hospital Grenoble, Grenoble, France

Chapter 1

Pharmacology of High-Dose Buprenorphine

Pierre Marquet

1. INTRODUCTION

Buprenorphine is a semisynthetic opioid derived from thebaine, an alcaloid of the poppy *Papaver somniferum*. Alan Cowan and John Lewis first synthesized buprenorphine in the United States in 1973 and also described its main properties, including its potential efficacy as a substitution treatment for heroin *(1)*.

Buprenorphine is a very lipid-soluble molecule ($\log Kp > 3$), with a mol wt of 467.65 Da, a first pKa of 8.42, and a second of 9.83. Its chemical structure, presented in Fig. 1., shows the same skeleton as morphine but with higher lipid solubility owing to the presence of two nonpolar sidechains. This molecule presents pharmacokinetic and pharmacodynamic peculiarities explaining buprenorphine's special administration route as well as its status as a maintenance treatment for heroin addicts.

In this chapter, I essentially present the pharmacokinetic and pharmacodynamic properties of buprenorphine. I only briefly cite the resulting administration modes and clinical effects because these makeup the main core of the book and are discussed in detail later.

2. PHARMACOKINETIC PROPERTIES

2.1. Absorption and Bioavailability

Buprenorphine, being very lipid soluble, is well absorbed by the digestive route but presents a low bioavailability (<20%) by this route owing to a strong intestinal and hepatic first-pass effect. Therefore, oral administration is

From *Forensic Science and Medicine: Buprenorphine Therapy of Opiate Addiction*
Edited by: P. Kintz and P. Marquet © Humana Press Inc., Totowa, NJ

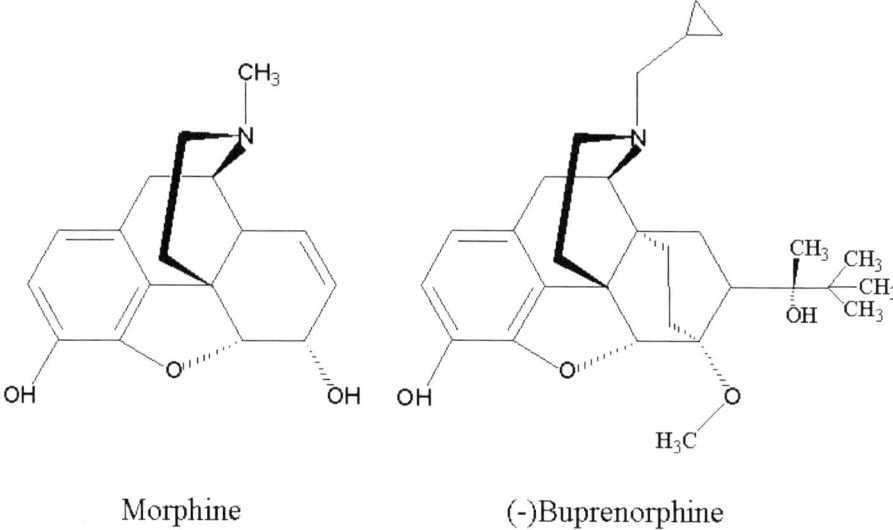

Fig. 1. Chemical structure of buprenorphine as compared with morphine.

not therapeutically convenient. By the transdermal route, insignificant blood levels are reached, even when using various buprenorphine esters, probably because the drug is sequestered in the lipid-rich skin layers *(2)*.

The bioavailability of buprenorphine by the sublingual (sl) route is greater and generally ranges between 30 and 55% *(3)*, but it is largely dependent on the time the drug is in contact with the oral mucosa *(4)*. On the other hand, several studies have demonstrated that the bioavailability was higher with liquid formulations of buprenorphine than with tablets *(5,6)*.

Linhardt et al. *(7)* even investigated the intranasal route: sheep were given low-dose buprenorphine and showed high bioavailability by this route (70–89%) with a short time to maximal concentration in plasma (T_{max} = 10 min on average) *(7)*. However, these investigators envisaged this route only for the treatment of pain. Indeed, daily intranasal administration in the long term might induce severe local side effects, even if buprenorphine is not a vasoconstrictor, as opposed to cocaine. Finally, sustained-release formulations of buprenorphine were also studied, e.g., under the form of biodegradable microcapsules that could elicit monthly administration *(8)*.

As is already the case for low-dose buprenorphine in the treatment of pain, sl tablets is the formulation currently used in those countries where high-dose buprenorphine is commercialized. This choice is probably based on practical considerations as well as on an expected lower abuse potential than with liquid formulations. However, in France this expectation has been dashed, because permissive prescription on a large scale has resulted in a large black market in the drug.

2.2. Distribution

Here again, most of the processes involved in the distribution phase are governed by the high lipid solubility of buprenorphine. It is 96% bound to plasma globulins, and exhibits a relatively high distribution volume (about 2.5 L/kg) and long distribution half-life (2–5 h). It is first distributed to the lipid-rich organs and tissues with a large blood supply (mainly brain and liver). Then it is redistributed from these tissues to body fat, which has a smaller blood supply but for which the drug presents a high affinity.

Buprenorphine readily and rapidly crosses the blood-brain barrier, which translates as much higher brain than plasma levels. For the standard doses used for maintenance treatment, only buprenorphine can be found in the brains of deceased patients, even when buprenorphine is suspected to be the cause of or a favoring factor in death, which means that the main metabolites do not cross the blood-brain barrier and that buprenorphine is not metabolized in the brain. This was confirmed in animal studies in which very high doses of buprenorphine and norbuprenorphine were administered intravenously (Fig. 2) *(9)*. However, in a case of suicide by ingestion of an extremely high dose of buprenorphine, we found a very high concentration of norbuprenorphine as well as buprenorphine in brain tissue, suggesting an increase in the permeability of the blood-brain barrier or maybe an overloading of a hypothetical rejection mechanism by a transport protein such as P-glycoprotein *(10)*.

Buprenorphine is incorporated into hair. Hair growth is approx 1 cm/mo, so hair analysis might help evaluate compliance in maintenance patients. However, such hair analyses have limitations for therapeutic drug monitoring or even compliance assessment, as shown by a retrospective study in six male and six female volunteers administered 8 mg/d of buprenorphine sublingually for 40–180 d *(11)*. Although buprenorphine and norbuprenorphine were generally detectable in the hair, these molecules, in some volunteers, were detected in hair segments (1 cm long) corresponding to a period of time anterior to the treatment, suggesting molecule movements in the hair shaft or external contamination by sweat (the mechanisms generally proposed for xenobiotic incorporation into hair are internal diffusion of compounds from blood toward hair follicle cells and external diffusion from sweat or sebaceous secretion toward the hair shaft). That study also showed a very high variability in the concentrations measured of different individuals prescribed the same dose. Moreover, in one of them buprenorphine and norbuprenorphine were not found in any of the hair segments, but drug administration was not controlled, which

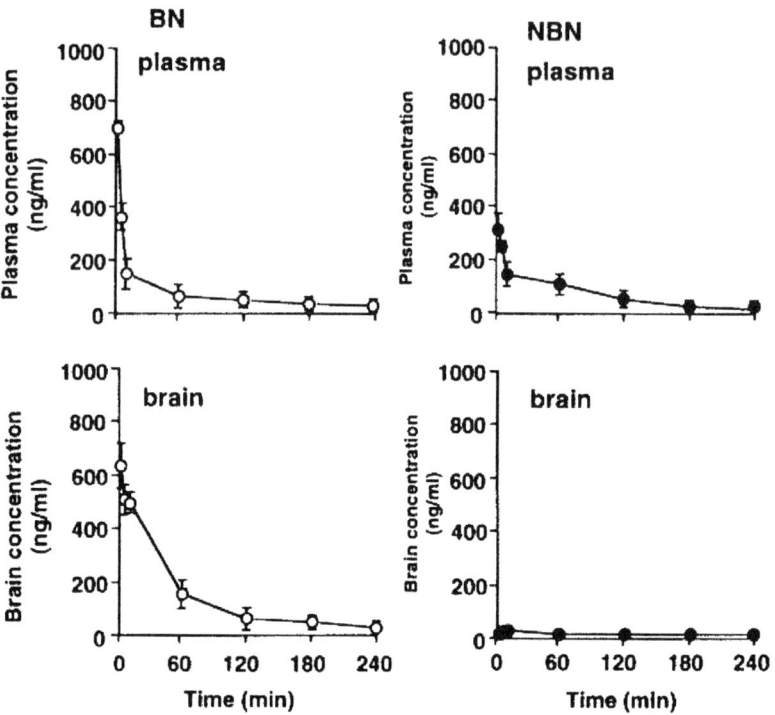

Fig. 2. Mean plasma and brain concentration time profile of buprenorphine (BN) and norbuprenorphine (NBN) after IV injection of 0.6 mg/kg of buprenorphine and 0.6 mg/kg of norbuprenorphine into three rats. (From ref. 23 with permission.)

is also a limitation for the interpretation of the other findings of that study. However, it seems clear that hair analysis cannot be used for buprenorphine dose adaptation in maintenance patients. Finally, the norbuprenorphine-to-buprenorphine ratio seems to vary a lot as a function of the method used to decontaminate hair and to extract these molecules from the hair matrix (12,13). Most of the researchers found higher concentrations of the metabolite in hair of patients chronically dosed, whereas, generally, parent compounds, which are more lipid soluble, are better incorporated into hair than their metabolites. This could be an artifact because the decontamination procedures by organic solvents employed could wash away a much larger quantity of buprenorphine than norbuprenorphine (13). Such an artifact might also have interfered with the results of the aforementioned clinical study.

2.3. Metabolism

Buprenorphine is mainly metabolized in the intestinal wall and the liver, first by a dealkylation reaction catalyzed by cytochrome P450 3A4, leading to norbuprenorphine *(14)*, then by glucuroconjugation of buprenorphine and norbuprenorphine. Clinically, norbuprenorphine appears to be weakly active, whereas the glucuronides appear to be inactive. Metabolism of buprenorphine is moderately affected in hepatic failure. Moreover, buprenorphine weakly inhibits CYP 3A4 in vitro *(15)* and shows no pharmacokinetic interaction with flunitrazepam *(16)*. This gives little consistency to the hypothesis of an accumulation of benzodiazepine in the numerous lethal cases in which the association high-dose buprenorphine-benzodiazepines was reported, as further demonstrated by the often "therapeutic" blood levels of benzodiazepine found *(17,18)*.

2.4. Excretion

Ninety percent of the administered dose is eliminated via the bile, essentially in the form of buprenorphine and norbuprenorphine glucuronides; bile concentrations are much higher than plasma concentrations *(10,17)*. After hydrolysis of the glucuronides by the intestinal flora, free buprenorphine and norbuprenorphine enter enterohepatic circulation *(19)*. A part of the administered dose is also eliminated in the urine, mainly as glucuronides and, to a lesser extent, norbuprenorphine then buprenorphine, all of which can be found in this fluid for several days after the last dose. The terminal half-life of buprenorphine is on average 20–25 h, corresponding to the return of buprenorphine and norbuprenorphine from tissue storage (particularly body fat) to the vascular compartment.

Nevertheless, probably owing to its large distribution volume, the steady-state, trough blood level of buprenorphine is very low (on the order of 1–10 ng/mL for a daily sl dose of 4–16 mg), requiring sensitive analytical techniques, and presents a large interindividual as well as, but to a lesser extent, intraindividual variability. However, the plasma level, whether peak or trough, increases with the dose *(20)*.

3. PHARMACODYNAMIC PROPERTIES

Buprenorphine has a variable affinity for and intrinsic activity on the different opioid receptor types. Its affinity for the μ receptors, the endogenous ligands of which are β-endorphin and, to a lesser extent, Met-enkephalin and dynorphins, is roughly 2000 times that of morphine. Moreover, buprenorphine very slowly dissociates from these receptors, exhibiting a fixation half-life of approx 40 min (vs milliseconds for morphine), which is responsible for its prolonged effects. Buprenorphine is only a partial agonist for these receptors, meaning that its maximal effect is lower than that of morphine, which is called a *ceiling effect (21,22)*. This very high affinity and the ceiling effect explain why buprenorphine can act as a relative competitive antagonist for morphine. On the other hand, by stimulating these μ receptors, buprenorphine induces clinical effects similar to those of morphine: analgesia, euphoria, but also respiratory depression and dependence. Its metabolite norbuprenorphine exerts a weak intrinsic activity on μ receptors *(23)* in vivo. Ohtani et al. *(9)* compared the effects of increasing doses of buprenorphine and norbuprenorphine administered by IV bolus infusion in animals (1–3 mg/kg). The analgesic effect of norbuprenorphine was about 50 times less than that of buprenorphine, whereas norbuprenorphine was much more prone to induce respiratory depression (at 0.008–3 mg/kg), as demonstrated by a decrease in respiratory rate and an increase in arterial PCO_2 (Fig. 3). This was probably caused by stimulating lung μ receptors rather than the respiratory center in the brainstem, since intraarterial administration of the same doses showed no respiratory effects. Note that the doses administered in this study were much higher than those used in maintenance patients (about 0.05–0.3 mg/kg by the sublingual route). Moreover, the minimum respiratory rate was observed 15 min after iv dosing, which might suggest the effect of a metabolite produced in the lung (maybe norbuprenorphine-glucuronide, by analogy to the effects of morphine-6-glucuronide).

On κ receptors, whose endogenous ligands are dynorphins and β-endorphin, buprenorphine activity is complex: it is an antagonist of $κ_2$ receptors, which are responsible for the dysphoria exerted by other opiates such as etorphine or pentazocine *(24)*. Together with butorphanol, buprenorphine would thus be the most selective agonist-antagonist for μ and κ receptors, respectively *(25)*. However, buprenorphine is an agonist of the $κ_1$ and $κ_3$ subtypes, which would reinforce its analgesic potency *(26)*, particularly at the spinal level *(24)*.

Buprenorphine has a very weak affinity for δ receptors (whose endogenous ligands are mainly enkephalins and β-endorphin), which would explain the absence of a "high" feeling when administered.

A recent in vitro study showed that norbuprenorphine exhibited affinities for μ, κ, and δ receptors comparable with those of buprenorphine, and that it would be a potent partial agonist at μ and κ receptors and a potent full agonist of δ receptors *(27)*. These results are not inconsistent with the absence of clinical effects of norbuprenorphine, at least for usual doses of high-dose

Pharmacology of High-Dose Buprenorphine

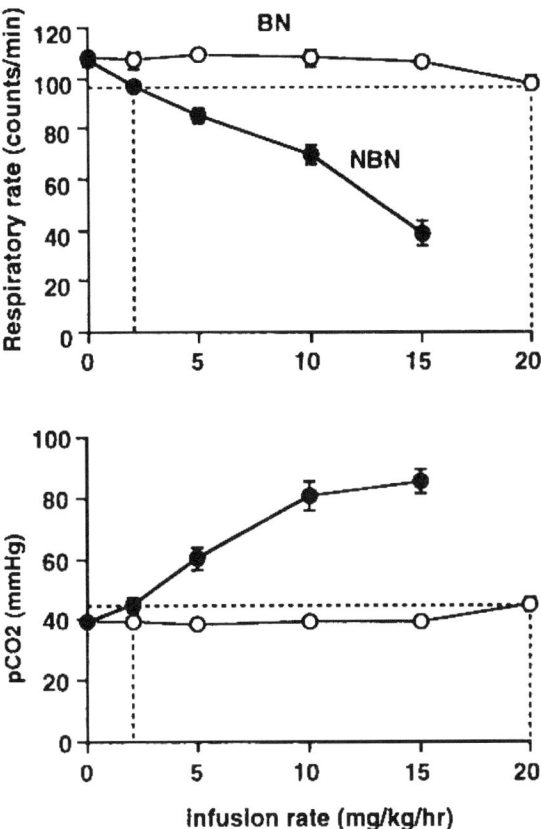

Fig. 3. Mean respiratory effects of buprenorphine (BN) and norbuprenorphine (NBN) in rats, as a function of infusion rate ($n = 3$). (From ref. 23 with permission.)

buprenorphine, because this metabolite does not seem to cross the blood-brain barrier, nor to be produced in the brain. However, they need to be confirmed using different in vitro as well as animal models.

In response to prolonged stimulation by high-dose buprenorphine, animal experiments showed a desensitization of μ receptors in the frontal cortex, thalamus, hippocampus, striatum, and brain stem, as well as an overexpression of k_1 receptors in the striatum and the frontal, parietal, and occipital cortex (28). However, this desensitization by receptor phosphorylation is minimal with respect to that induced by full agonists for these receptors (such as etorphine) or by morphine (29). On the other hand, this would not be the only or even the most important mechanism involved in opiate tolerance. Indeed, stimulation of opioid receptors, which are all coupled to G proteins, results in an inhibition of cellular adenylyl cyclase and therefore in a decrease in intracellular cAMP *(30)*. Prolonged administration of morphine but not buprenorphine or methadone *(31)* induces a marked increase in the expression of the G proteins, of several protein kinases, and above all of adenylyl cyclase, allowing cAMP to reach intracellular concentrations close to normal (i.e., in the absence of opioid stimulation), with even a rebound (high cAMP concentrations) when morphine is stopped *(30)*. However, these two different mechanisms could take place on different timescales, the latter within a few days or weeks and receptor desensitization in the longer term. Buprenorphine was shown to antagonize the μ receptor phosphorylation induced by morphine as well as to abolish the ability of opioids to inhibit adenylyl cyclase *(31)*.

4. Administration Schedules

In France, high-dose buprenorphine (Subutex®) is available as 0.4-, 2-, and 8-mg sl tablets, and the recommended administration scheme is once daily, based on the duration of the psychotropic effects of buprenorphine, which are linked to the stability of the buprenorphine-receptor complex rather than to the pharmacokinetic properties of buprenorphine. Numerous studies have even demonstrated the possibility of administering higher doses once every 2, 3, or 4 d *(32)*. These studies in maintenance patients, always conducted under controlled conditions, found an increase in the plasma concentration of buprenorphine as a function of the dose, without noticeable side effects. These results are in favor of less frequent dosing, which would mean less frequent visits for the patients to the maintenance centers and thus probably an increase in the treatment capacity of these centers.

High-dose buprenorphine has even been tested for detoxification of heroin addicts, owing to the mild withdrawal syndromes it induces and its property of antagonizing the other opiates *(33)*. A review article has shown that all the studies comparing the efficacy of clonidine and buprenorphine in 10-d detoxification programs reported a less severe withdrawal syndrome with buprenorphine, with a success rate between 65 and 100%, depending on the criteria selected *(34)*.

5. Clinical Effects of Buprenorphine

Buprenorphine has been used at low doses for its analgesic properties for about 20 yr in more than 40 countries worldwide. Its use at high doses since 1996 in France confirmed its ceiling effect on subjective measurements and respiratory depression, whereas, in a given individual, plasma concentration increases linearly with the dose. Very high doses were even administered during clinical studies in humans, with practically no side effects. Consistent with the slow rate of receptor phosphorylation, the development of tolerance seems very slow and clinically insignificant. Withdrawal syndromes are generally late and of moderate intensity. Finally, even if high-dose buprenorphine induces no "high effect" when administered sublingually, owing to its weak affinity for the δ receptors but also to a relatively slow delivery to the brain, it is apparently different with IV high-dose buprenorphine, which probably explains frequent abuse by this route in France (8% of maintenance patients or between 10 and 20%, depending on the authors *[35]*). To avoid such abuse, the addition of naloxone to the sl preparation of high-dose buprenorphine is being studied, particularly in the United States. The rationale, interests, and potential drawbacks of this association are detailed in Chapter 4.

6. CONCLUSION

Buprenorphine is a semisynthetic opiate with partial agonist as well as antagonist properties for the different types of opioid receptors that exerts analgesic effects, moderate respiratory depression, no hallucinations, and no "high" feeling when administered sublingually and has a protracted maintenance potential. The "ceiling" of its maximal effect provides this drug with a large security margin *when used alone*. On the contrary, its association with other psychotropic drugs would potentiate its respiratory depressant effects and lead to death in certain circumstances, as reported in Chapter 8.

REFERENCES

1. Cowan A, Lewis JW, Macfarlane IR. Agonist and antagonist properties of buprenorphine, a new antinociceptive agent. Br J Pharmacol 1977;60:537–45.
2. Stinchcomb AL, Paliwal A, Dua R, Imoto H, Woodard RW, Flynn GL. Permeation of buprenorphine and its 3–alkyl-ester prodrugs through human skin. Pharm Res 1996;13:1519–23.
3. Kuhlman JJ Jr, Lalani S, Magluilo J Jr, Levine B, Darwin WD. Human pharmacokinetics of intravenous, sublingual, and buccal buprenorphine. J Anal Toxicol 1996;20:369–78.
4. Mendelson J, Upton RA, Everhart ET, Jacob P III, Jones RT. Bioavailability of sublingual buprenorphine. J Clin Pharmacol 1997;37:31–7.
5. Nath RP, Upton RA, Everhart ET, Cheung P, Shwonek P, Jones RT, Mendelson JE. Buprenorphine pharmacokinetics: relative bioavailability of sublingual tablet and liquid formulations. J Clin Pharmacol 1999;39:619–23.
6. Schuh KJ, Johanson CE. Pharmacokinetic comparison of the buprenorphine sublingual liquid and tablet. Drug Alcohol Depend 1999;56:55–60.

7. Linhardt K, Ravn C, Gizurarson S, Bechgaard E. Intranasal absorption of buprenorphine—in vivo bioavailability in sheep. Int J Pharm 2000;205(1–2):159–63.
8. Mandal TK. Development of biodegradable drug delivery system to treat addiction. Drug Dev Ind Pharm 1999;25(6):773–9.
9. Ohtani M, Kotaki H, Nishitateno K, Sawada Y, Iga T. Kinetics of respiratory depression in rats induced by buprenorphine and its metabolite, norbuprenorphine. J Pharmacol Exp Ther 1997;281:428–33.
10. Gaulier JM, Marquet P, Lacassie E, Dupuy JL, Lachatre G. Fatal intoxication following self-administration of a massive dose of buprenorphine. J Forensic Sci 2000;45:226–8.
11. Wilkins DG, Rollins DE, Valdez AS, Mizuno A, Krueger GG, Cone EJ. A retrospective study of buprenorphine and norbuprenorphine in human hair after multiple doses. J Anal Toxicol 1999;23(6);409–5.
12. Vincent F, Bessard J, Vacheron J, Mallaret M, Bessard G. Determination of buprenorphine and norbuprenorphine in urine and hair by gas chromatography-mass spectrometry. J Anal Toxicol 1999;23(4):270–9.
13. Cirimele V, Kintz P, Lohner S, Ludes B. Buprenorphine to norbuprenorphine ratio in human hair. J Anal Toxicol 2000;24(6):448–9.
14. Iribarne C, Picart D, Dreano Y, Bail JP, Berthou F. Involvement of cytochrome P450 3A4 in N-dealkylation of buprenorphine in human liver microsomes. Life Sci 1997;60:1953–64.
15. Ibrahim RB, Wilson JG, Thorsby ME, Edwards DJ. Effect of buprenorphine on CYP3A activity in rat and human liver microsomes. Life Sci 2000;66:1293–8.
16. Kilicarslan T, Sellers EM. Lack of interaction of buprenorphine with flunitrazepam metabolism. Am J Psychiatry 2000;157:1164–6.
17. Tracqui A, Kintz P, Ludes B. Buprenorphine-related deaths among drug addicts in France: a report on 20 fatalities. J Anal Toxicol 1998;22(6):430–4.
18. Kintz P. Deaths involving buprenorphine: a compendium of French cases. Forensic Sci Int 2001;121:65–9.
19. Ohtani M, Kotaki H, Uchino K, Sawada Y, Iga T. Pharmacokinetic analysis of enterohepatic circulation of buprenorphine and its active metabolite, norbuprenorphine, in rats. Drug Metab Dispos 1994;22(1):2–7.
20. Chawarski MC, Schottenfeld RS, O'Connor PG, Pakes J. Plasma concentrations of buprenorphine 24 to 72 hours after dosing. Drug Alcohol Depend 1999;55(1–2):157–163.
21. Walsh SL, Preston KL, Stitzer ML, Cone EJ, Bigelow GE. Clinical pharmacology of buprenorphine: ceiling effects at high doses. Clin Pharmacol Ther 1994;55:569–80.
22. Walker EA, Zernig G, Young AM. In vivo apparent affinity and efficacy estimates for mu opiates in a rat tail-withdrawal assay. Psychopharmacology (Berl) 1998;136(1):15–23.
23. Ohtani M, Kotaki H, Sawada Y, Iga T. Comparative analysis of buprenorphine- and norbuprenorphine-induced analgesic effects based on pharmacokinetic-pharmacodynamic modeling. J Pharmacol Exp Ther 1995;272:505–10.
24. Rang HP, Dale MM, Ritter JM. Pharmacology, 4th ed., Churchill Livingstone, Edinburgh, UK; 1999.

25. Ohta S, Niwa M, Nozaki M, Hattori M, Shimonaka H, Dohi S. The mu, delta and kappa properties of various opioids. Masui 1995;44(9):1228–32.
26. Pick CG, Peter Y, Schreiber S, Weizman R. Pharmacological characterization of buprenorphine, a mixed agonist-antagonist with kappa 3 analgesia. Brain Res 1997;744:41–6.
27. Huang P, Kehner GB, Cowan A, Liu-Chen LY. Comparison of pharmacological activities of buprenorphine and norbuprenorphine: norbuprenorphine is a potent opioid agonist. J Pharmacol Exp Ther 2001;297:688–95.
28. Belcheva MM, Ho MT, Igantova EG, Jefcoat LB, Barg J, Vogel Z, McHale RJ, Johnson FE, Coscia CJ. Buprenorphine differentially alters opioid receptor adaptation in rat brain regions. J Pharmacol Exp Ther 1996;277:1322–7.
29. Yu Y, Zhang L, Yi X, Sun H, Uhl GR, Wang JB. Mu opioid receptor phosphorylation, desensitization and ligand efficacy. J Biol Chem 1997; 272: 28,869–74.
30. Sharma SK, Nirenberg M, Klee WA. Morphine receptors as regulators of adenylate cyclase activity. Proc Natl Acad Sci USA 1975;72(2):590–4.
31. Blake AD, Bot G, Freeman JC, Reisine T. Differential opioid agonist regulation of the mouse µ opioid receptor. JBC 1997;272(2):782–90.
32. Petry NM, Bickel WK, Badger GJ. A comparison of four buprenophine dosing regimens in the treatment of opioid dependence. Clin Pharmacol Ther 1999;66: 306–14.
33. Vignau J. Preliminary assessment of a 10–day rapid detoxification programme using high dosage buprenorphine. Eur Addict Res 1998;4 Suppl 1:29–31.
34. Gowing L, Ali R, White J. Buprenorphine for the management of opioid withdrawal. Cochrane Database Syst Rev 2000;3:CD002025.
35. Pratiques en évolution: bonnes pratiques de prise en charge des pharmaco-dépendances majeures aux opiacés. Ed. Schering-Plough, Levallois Perret;1999.

Chapter 2

Controlled Drug Administration Studies of High-Dose Buprenorphine in Humans

Marilyn A. Huestis

1. INTRODUCTION

Buprenorphine was developed in the early 1970s by Reckitt and Colman Products (Hull, UK) as part of a wide-ranging search for an effective analgesic with lower abuse potential and reduced toxicity compared with morphine *(1)*. Many of buprenorphine's chemical and pharmacological properties, including ready diffusion of the highly lipophilic drug across the blood-brain barrier and its high binding avidity for opiate receptors, led to the selection of this thebaine derivative as the best analgesic compound for further drug development. Despite its high-affinity binding and high potency (25–40 times more potent than morphine), buprenorphine has a lower efficacy for pain relief and is classified as a partial agonist at μ opiate receptors. Buprenorphine dissociates slowly from receptors, resulting in a long duration of action and, potentially, a reduced potential for abuse. These properties led researchers at the United States Public Health Service's Addiction Research Center to investigate buprenorphine further as a pharmacotherapy for opioid addiction *(2)*.

Several important factors need to be considered when reviewing the buprenorphine literature. Over the last 25 yr, investigators have studied the agonist and antagonist characteristics of buprenorphine alone and its interactions when coadministered with other opioids. Buprenorphine may substitute for another opioid, suppress response to an opioid, or precipitate withdrawal from an opioid, depending on the dose of buprenorphine administered and conditions at the time of administration. Careful consideration must be given

From *Forensic Science and Medicine: Buprenorphine Therapy of Opiate Addiction*
Edited by: P. Kintz and P. Marquet © Humana Press Inc., Totowa, NJ

to participant drug use history, frequency, magnitude and length of opioid use, buprenorphine dosing regimen, and the nature of studied effects, for all of these parameters can affect the interpretation of research findings. In addition, evaluation of buprenorphine concentration data requires an understanding of the sensitivity and specificity of the analytical method employed. Much of the early buprenorphine literature utilized a highly sensitive but nonspecific radioimmunoassay (RIA) that crossreacted extensively with buprenorphine metabolites. At the time, chromatographic methods could not meet the sensitivity requirements mandated by the low concentrations of buprenorphine and metabolites found in plasma.

This chapter reviews controlled drug administration studies of buprenorphine in humans and focuses primarily on its use as a pharmacotherapeutic agent for opioid dependence, but important findings from analgesic research are included when appropriate. It examines buprenorphine's bioavailability following alternative routes of drug administration, dose effect profiles, abuse liability, and toxicity. The reader is referred to additional discussions on buprenorphine's efficacy as a replacement maintenance medication in opioid addiction treatment and buprenorphine poisonings in medical examiner cases included in later chapters of this book.

2. BIOAVAILABILITY

Intravenous (im) buprenorphine for analgesia was released for the treatment of moderate to severe pain in 1977. The oral route of drug administration was not pursued because substantial first-pass metabolism of buprenorphine led to limited oral bioavailability of approx 15% *(3)*. Extensive hepatic oxidative metabolism of buprenorphine by the cytochrome P450 3A4 isoenzyme was shown to produce the *n*-dealkylated metabolite, norbuprenorphine, a weak μ agonist with limited ability to penetrate the blood-brain barrier *(4)*. Therefore, a sublingual (sl) preparation for use in cancer patients unable to tolerate the oral route because of nausea and vomiting and the parenteral route because of poor venous access, emaciation, or coagulation defects was also made available. The sublingual or buccal route of buprenorphine administration also avoided first-pass metabolism, minimized side effects owing to lower peak drug concentrations (i.e., sedation and constipation), and allowed rapid drug absorption owing to a high lipid to water partition coefficient *(5)*. Disadvantages of the sl route include an unpalatable taste, mucosal irritation, and large intersubject variability.

Early pharmacokinetic studies by Bullingham et al. *(6)* observed maximum plasma concentrations (C_{max}) approx 3 h after sl administration of 0.4

and 0.8 mg of buprenorphine with an absorption half-life of 76 min. A good dose-concentration relationship was noted at these low doses, and sl bioavailability was found to be approximately 55% based on the nonspecific RIA *(7)*. Weinberg et al. *(8)* reported rapid absorption of sl buprenorphine into the oral mucosa, but a slower absorption from this tissue reservoir of drug into the systemic circulation. Buprenorphine absorption via the sl route at these low doses was found to be dose independent with maximal absorption into the oral mucosa by 2.5 min. In addition, the duration of action of sl buprenorphine was found to be longer than that found after equianalgesic doses of iv or im preparations, most likely owing to an available reservoir of drug in the oral mucosa. Further evidence for a mucosal reservoir of drug was noted by Cone et al. *(9)*, who reported elevated salivary buprenorphine concentrations for up to 12 h in subjects treated with sl buprenorphine, in contrast to low salivary concentrations following im administration. Equivalent plasma and saliva concentrations of buprenorphine were not realized until 24–48 h after the end of chronic sl dosing.

Buprenorphine is a highly lipophilic compound that accumulates in the tissues to a much higher extent than in blood with chronic dosing *(10)*. This tissue depot contributes to the long terminal elimination half-life (42 h) of the drug and suggested that transdermal delivery of buprenorphine could, perhaps, be a feasible route of drug administration for chronic pain *(11)*. Effective analgesia has been achieved with transdermal buprenorphine, although a lag time of 1–6 h was observed even with an ethanol-based delivery device *(12,13)*. Attempts to deliver drug via the transdermal route in concentrations sufficient for treatment of opioid dependence were unsuccessful *(14)*.

The long half-life of buprenorphine and strong binding to opiate receptors led Fudala et al. *(15)* to evaluate the effectiveness of alternate-day administration of buprenorphine in the treatment of opioid addiction. Although subjects had a significantly greater urge for opioids on days when they did not receive buprenorphine, they were able to tolerate 48 h between doses. In addition, only mild to moderate opioid withdrawal symptoms developed following abrupt termination of drug after chronic treatment. Peak effects on the Himmelsbach withdrawal scale occurred after 3–5 d of abstinence and lasted for up to 10 d. These data indicate that the combined factors of an extended plasma half-life for buprenorphine and accumulated drug stored in the tissues following chronic dosing provide sufficient drug concentration to allow alternate-day drug administration and to delay the onset of severe withdrawal symptoms.

Tablet sl formulations offer advantages over liquid ones including increased drug stability, ease of storage, simplified drug administration, and reduced potential for accidental ingestion by children. Mendelson et al. *(16,17)* evaluated absorption of sl buprenorphine from tablets containing 4–32 mg of drug alone and in combination with naloxone. The mean buprenorphine area under the curve (AUC) and C_{max} were found to increase with increasing dose, but dose-corrected AUC was lower for each increase in dose. These findings are in disagreement with those found with the liquid sl preparation, indicating a possible difference in absorption between the liquid and tablet sl formulations. A ceiling on sl buprenorphine absorption may occur with the tablet formulation and may contribute to observed ceiling effects on buprenorphine opioid agonist effects when tablets are administered. Later studies determined bioavailability of buprenorphine from the sl tablet to be approx 50% that of the liquid sl formulation *(18,19)*.

3. DOSE-EFFECT PROFILES

Buprenorphine has a bell-shaped dose-response curve. Early studies demonstrated a lack of orderly dose effect responses for pain relief after 0.2–0.8 mg of sl buprenorphine *(20)*, for euphoria following 0.2–2 mg of subcutaneous (sc) buprenorphine *(2)*, and for respiratory depression following 0.3 and 0.6 mg of iv buprenorphine *(3,21)*. Because studies documenting the success of buprenorphine in reducing heroin use and increasing retention of patients in opioid treatment programs also suggested that higher doses of sl buprenorphine could improve treatment outcomes *(22–24)*, Walsh et al. *(25)* studied the safety, tolerability, and abuse liability of up to 32 mg of sl buprenorphine in opioid-experienced but nondependent volunteers. Subjective effects and respiratory depression failed to increase in a dose proportional manner with higher sl buprenorphine doses. Maximal effects were always reached prior to the highest 32-mg dose. Despite increases in plasma buprenorphine concentrations with higher sl doses, behavioral and physiological responses did not increase, documenting that the observed ceiling effect was not owing to limited sl absorption. Another important observation from this study was the increased duration of action noted after high sl doses. Euphoria and miosis lasted up to 3 d after a single acute 32-mg sl dose of buprenorphine. The investigators suggested that the lower efficacy of buprenorphine at higher doses could reduce the risk of overdose and perhaps its abuse liability, increasing the safety of buprenorphine maintenance therapy.

4. ABUSE LIABILITY

Heroin, morphine, and other semisynthetic opioids produce μ-agonist reinforcing effects sometimes leading to self-administration and physical dependence owing to their high potential for abuse liability. Treatment of iv heroin dependence reduces the health and social consequences of drug addiction, the transmission of infectious diseases including the human immunodeficiency virus (HIV), and drug-related criminal activity. Pharmacotherapy for opiate addiction, especially in conjunction with behavioral treatment, reduces drug use. Methadone, levomethadyl acetate, and naltrexone are approved opioid agonist and antagonist treatments for opioid addiction in the United States. Opioid agonist replacement medications are currently only available from a few highly regulated treatment programs. Patients are required to receive daily or alternate-day medications under observed conditions except when they have demonstrated significant progress in their treatment and earned the privilege of occasional "take-home" doses. This stringent control on medications is needed to prevent drug diversion and iv self-administration. The search continues for additional useful medications with low abuse potential that would allow patients to obtain needed treatment more readily.

Buprenorphine is one of the most promising new analgesics. A partial agonist at μ opiate receptors, buprenorphine can antagonize the euphoria produced by other opiates. It also has a long duration of action and decreased physical dependence following chronic treatment. However, buprenorphine does produce morphine-like subjective feelings, increasing the potential for drug diversion and abuse.

Jasinski et al. *(2)* first suggested that buprenorphine be used as a maintenance drug for opioid dependence. Buprenorphine's abuse potential was found to be limited with less euphoria at higher sc doses. Furthermore, its long half-life prevented the onset of withdrawal until 14 d after the last dose of buprenorphine following 30–57 daily doses of 8 mg subcutaneously. Withdrawal symptoms were found to be mild and lasted only a few days. These characteristics suggested that daily or less frequent dosing could be effective in buprenorphine treatment of addicts. A substantial potential for abuse of buprenorphine by the iv route was noted in a study assessing the subjective effects of 0.3, 0.6, and 1.2 mg of iv buprenorphine in nondependent opiate users *(26)*. Intravenous buprenorphine produced positive responses on reliable predictors of abuse liability including "feel drug" questionnaires and increased drug "liking," "good effects," and euphoria scores (as measured by the morphine benzedrine [MBG] scale of the Addiction Research Center Inventory [ARCI]).

One of the important factors in selecting a therapeutic medication for opiate dependence is the drug's acceptability to patients. Naltrexone is an effective opioid antagonist and useful in the treatment of addiction, but it is disliked by many opiate abusers and compliance to treatment has been poor *(27,28)*. Buprenorphine produces increases in positive subjective effects, albeit at a lower magnitude than full µ agonists. Up to 4 mg of sl buprenorphine and up to 2 mg of sc buprenorphine were observed to produce varying degrees of euphoria with increased subject-reported drug-liking scores *(29)*. Study participants identified the drug as opiate-like and reported little dysphoria and sedation. Administration of sl buprenorphine was shown to delay the onset of reinforcing effects as compared to iv administration, reducing its abuse potential. An sl drug delivery system was recommended for treatment of opioid dependence to reduce illicit drug diversion (compared to injectable drug), to reduce manufacturing cost (compared to oral preparations that have more limited bioavailability), and to facilitate drug administration as compared to the sc route.

Illicit use of buprenorphine by the iv route may become especially problematic when heroin cost is high and its supply unreliable *(30–32)*. A creative approach to the problem of potential diversion of therapeutic buprenorphine has been the addition of naloxone, a µ opiate antagonist, to the medication. An im combination of 0.3 mg of buprenorphine and 0.2 mg of naloxone provided good analgesic relief, similar to buprenorphine alone, with only a slightly delayed time of onset. The bioavailability of sl naloxone was estimated to be approx 30%, thus providing some antagonism to buprenorphine's effects at this low agonist:antagonist ratio. Plasma concentrations of naloxone after the oral route are close to zero owing to extensive first-pass metabolism *(8)*.

Preston et al. *(34)* evaluated physiological and behavioral effects of buprenorphine and naloxone alone and in different combinations in opioid-dependent humans. Subcutaneous buprenorphine alone (0.2 and 0.3 mg) produced no significant effects on any measure, whereas sc naloxone alone (0.2 mg) precipitated abstinence. The sc combinations of 0.2 mg of buprenorphine and 0.2 mg of naloxone, and sc 0.3 mg of buprenorphine and 0.2 mg of naloxone sc also produced an attenuated withdrawal, suggesting a lower abuse potential for the combination product.

Combinations of im buprenorphine and naloxone were also tested in nondependent opioid abusers *(35)*. Buprenorphine alone produced dose-related opioid agonist effects on physiological and subjective measures. When administered with similar concentrations of naloxone (0.4 mg/70 kg of buprenorphine and 0.5 mg/70 kg of naloxone), opioid agonist effects were attenuated; higher ratios of naloxone:buprenorphine resulted in complete attenuation of opioid effects. The combination product was recommended as a means of lowering the abuse liability of buprenorphine alone, similar to the reduction in abuse of pentazocine-naloxone tablets. In another study in eight opiate-experienced volunteers, naloxone, in a 1:4 ratio with buprenorphine, did not alter sl buprenorphine pharmacokinetics or pharmacodynamic effects and did not produce opioid withdrawal *(16)*.

5. TOXICITY

Opiates, such as morphine and heroin, produce respiratory depression in a dose-related manner. Although parenteral buprenorphine also was shown to decrease responsiveness to increasing plasma carbon dioxide concentrations, this effect was much less than that seen following morphine *(36)*. Further support for the high therapeutic index of buprenorphine was found in the lack of clinically relevant respiratory effects in individuals receiving up to 16 mg/d of sl buprenorphine for 84 d while participating in an opioid replacement research protocol *(37)*. The maximum observed decrease in respiratory rate was two breaths per minute at the highest dose of buprenorphine.

In 1979, in one of the first reported buprenorphine overdose cases, it was noted that ingestion of approx forty 0.4-mg buprenorphine tablets by the sl or oral route (the route could not be definitively identified) produced minimal drowsiness and no respiratory or hemodynamic disturbances *(38)*. The partial agonist action of buprenorphine and reduced bioavailability by the oral and sl routes may account for this limited toxicity *(39,40)*. In a study of nondependent healthy individuals *(41)*, respiratory rate and oxygen saturation were found to be minimally affected following 8 mg of sl buprenorphine. Furthermore, up to 7 mg of parenteral buprenorphine produced no clinically significant respiratory depression in 50 female cesarian section patients who received the drug for analgesia *(42)*. In fact, respiratory depression was rarely found to be significant, except when used together with other depressants, especially benzodiazepines, during surgery *(43–46)*.

Zanette et al. *(47)* report a serious case of buprenorphine interaction involving an 11-yr-old female who developed severe and prolonged respiratory depression following administration of 4 µg/kg of im buprenorphine 12 h after surgery for relief of pain and restlessness. Her respiration had been stable after a successful surgical procedure that utilized diazepam, fentanyl, and other drugs for anesthesia. However, while in the intensive care unit, an additional 10 mg of diazepam was administered, reinstituting full respiratory insufficiency. The authors of this report warn of the dangers of coadministration of multiple sedative drugs. Respiratory and cardiovascular collapse has been reported in patients receiving therapeutic doses of buprenorphine and diazepam *(48)*. Reports from France, where high-dose buprenorphine has been available since 1996 for opioid maintenance treatment, indicate that physicians may be putting patients at risk by not following suggested dosing recommendations and continuing to coprescribe buprenorphine and benzodiazepines *(49)*.

The interaction between buprenorphine and benzodiazapines may be the result of pharmacokinetic or pharmacodynamics effects. In an in vitro investigation of the interaction of buprenorphine and benzodiazepines with Cyp3A enzymes from rat and human microsomes, Ibrahim et al. *(50)* found that the observed enzyme inhibition at typical plasma concentrations of benzodiazepine was unlikely to be responsible for excessive central nervous system (CNS) depression. An additive or synergistic pharmacological effect, unrelated to the pharmacokinetic interaction, was suggested as the cause of decreased respiratory function.

Interactions between the antidepressant amitriptyline and buprenorphine have also been reported; antidepressants may be commonly coprescribed with analgesics especially when chronic pain is accompanied by depression *(51)*. Sublingual buprenorphine alone depressed respiration, but a significant increase in end-tidal carbon dioxide was noted 2–4 h after coadministration of amitriptyline and buprenorphine. Concurrent administration of selective serotonin reuptake inhibitor antidepressants (e.g., fluvoxamine) has also been shown to increase the bioavailability of buprenorphine owing to noncompetitive inhibition of the P450 3A4 isoenzyme *(52)*. HIV-1 protease inhibitors, ritonavir and indinavir, also competitively inhibit n-dealkylation of buprenorphine *(53)*. Cyp 3A4 represents about 30% of the total P450 content of the human liver; many licit and illicit drugs are known to induce or inhibit these enzymes and, hence, buprenorphine metabolism. Thus, the observed toxicity of buprenorphine and other medications may be the result of complex pharmacokinetic and pharmacodynamic interactions.

High concentrations of norbuprenorphine may also contribute to buprenorphine toxicity. Utilizing extracted and unextracted samples and two different RIA antisera, Hand et al. *(54)* were able to estimate buprenorphine and metabolite concentrations after chronic dosing. Plasma concentrations of norbuprenorphine were low after single doses of buprenorphine, but equivalent to parent drug concentrations after daily dosing. Two- to threefold higher concentrations of buprenorphine glucuronide, the primary product of phase II metabolism, were found with chronic dosing. Although norbuprenorphine is much less potent than buprenorphine in producing analgesia, Ohrani et al. *(55)* have recently reported its higher respiratory depressant potency (10 times that of the parent drug). Increased plasma concentrations of norbuprenorphine may therefore, contribute to buprenorphine toxicity, although its ability to enter the brain is limited. Ohtani et al. *(55)* suggest that norbuprenorphine binding to μ receptors in the lung could account for its respiratory effects or

High-Dose Buprenorphine in Humans

that multiple μ receptor subtypes associated with analgesia or respiratory depression could bind with different affinities to buprenorphine and norbuprenorphine.

More than 70% of a buprenorphine dose is eliminated in the feces; renal clearance is much less important for drug clearance. Therefore, administration of buprenorphine may be advantageous over other analgesics when renal insufficiency is present. However, increased concentrations of the metabolites, free and conjugated norbuprenorphine and buprenorphine glucuronide, can increase dramatically when renal function is reduced. Poor renal function could lead to higher norbuprenorphine concentrations, increasing the potential for respiratory depression.

6. Safety and Abuse Liability of High-Dose Intravenous Buprenorphine

Concerns have been raised about the potential diversion and iv abuse of buprenorphine once it is approved for use in the United States. The safety and abuse liability of iv buprenorphine in the range of doses recommended for maintenance treatment have not been evaluated. In addition, although ceilings on physiological and subjective effects have been shown with high sl doses of buprenorphine, this phenomenon has not been tested at high iv doses. We (Clinical Pharmacology and Therapeutics Research Branch, NIDA) designed a protocol to determine the acute health risks of sl opioid maintenance doses if abused by the iv route, to evaluate the abuse liability of iv buprenorphine in nondependent iv opioid users, to characterize the effects of dose and time on behavior following high-dose iv buprenorphine, and to characterize the pharmacokinetics of buprenorphine and norbuprenorphine after iv administration *(56–59)*.

Sublingual buprenorphine (placebo or 12 mg) was held under the tongue for 5 min followed by iv buprenorphine administration of (placebo or 2, 4, 8, 12, or 16 mg) to six healthy male nondependent opioid users in this preliminary dose-escalation study. Physiological measures, including blood pressure (BP), heart rate, transcutaneous oxygen saturation, respiration rate, and skin temperature, were monitored continuously for 3 h and intermittently for 72 h after dosing. Visual analog scales for "any drug effects," "drug liking," "good effects," "bad effects," "high," "feel sick," and "desire opiates," an adjective rating scale; and a shortened form of the ARCI monitored subjective drug effects over the same time frame.

Intravenous administration of up to 16 mg of buprenorphine was shown to be safe in experienced, nondependent opioid abusers. It must be stressed that toxicity was minimal at these doses of buprenorphine alone. Combinations of buprenorphine and other compounds with respiratory depressant action have shown considerable toxicity. Various degrees of sedation, nausea, vomiting and itching were observed in participants in this study. Subjects were easily aroused with voice prompts and completed computer questionnaires and tasks throughout the experimental session. Some individuals became irritable after receiving these high iv doses of buprenorphine, but no other mental status changes were observed. One individual experienced severe nausea and vomiting after the 12-mg iv dose and did not participate in the highest 16-mg iv dose.

No significant differences from placebo in BP, heart rate, respiration rate, oxygen saturation, or skin temperature across time and drug conditions were noted (56). The only statistically significant difference was an increase in the 3-h AUC for systolic BP after the 8-mg iv dose (+13.5 mmHg). The mean (±SD) maximum decrease in oxygen saturation from baseline was −7.3% (±4.3) and was highest for the 8-mg iv dose.

All active buprenorphine conditions produced increases in positive subjective measures compared to placebo, including high, drug effect, good effects, drug liking, opioid agonist adjective rating scale, and MBG scale of the ARCI (56). Mean change from baseline scores ($n = 5$) for drug high as measured by Visual Analog Scale are shown for placebo, and for 2, 4, 8, 12, and 16 mg of iv buprenorphine in Fig. 1. Data are shown for the first 3 h after administration of drug. It is apparent that the strongest high effects were obtained following the 12-mg iv dose. Large interindividual differences in the magnitude of subjective effects were observed. Peak effects occurred 1–1.5 h after iv doses and 3–6 h after sl buprenorphine with a duration of action of 24–72 h. Effects did not increase in an orderly dose-related manner. On many measures, the magnitude of effect was not different between all active doses, consistent with a ceiling effect and partial agonist activity for buprenorphine. The effects of 16 mg intravenoulsy tended to be less than those of 12 mg and varied in comparison with other active doses. The effects of 12 mg sublingually were similar in magnitude to 4, 8, and 12 mg intravenously. The abuse potential of iv buprenorphine does not appear to increase with dose, nor does there appear to be a substantial difference in abuse potential between iv and sl buprenorphine at the doses tested.

Increases in subjective and physiological measures were not dose related and supported the presence of a ceiling effect for these parameters following iv administration. Plasma concentrations of buprenorphine and norbuprenorphine were also determined for up to 72 h after drug administration by liquid chromatography-tandem mass spectrometry. The limits of quantitation for buprenorphine and norbuprenorphine were 0.1 ng/mL utilizing deuterated

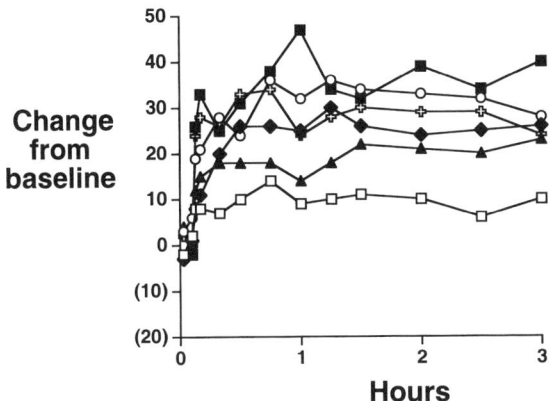

Fig. 1. Time course of mean change from baseline for drug high as measured with a Visual Analog Scale questionnaire ($n = 5$) following iv buprenorphine. Placebo (□), 2 (◆), 4 (○), 8 (▲), 12 (■), or 16 mg (⊕) iv buprenorphine was injected by a physician in a constant volume of 4 mL over 60 s to nondependent, opiate-experienced volunteers. Mean data for five of the six subjects are included because one subject in the trial did not receive the highest 16-mg in dose of buprenorphine.

internal standards for both analytes. Peak plasma concentrations of buprenorphine and norbuprenorphine occurred 0.5–2 h and 0.5–12 h after sl administration of drug. Peak plasma concentrations increased in an orderly dose-related manner suggesting that observed ceiling effects were owing to pharmacodynamic rather than pharmacokinetic factors. Doses were administered intravenously, ensuring that drug absorption was not a limiting factor.

Bioavailability following the sl route was determined to be approx 35%, in close agreement with another estimate obtained with a highly specific chromatographic method *(57)*. This is in contrast to earlier bioavailability estimates for sl buprenorphine of 55–65% that were based on nonspecific RIA measurements *(7)*.

7. Conclusion

Buprenorphine, a partial µ agonist and k antagonist, which is 25–40 times more potent than morphine, is an effective analgesic and opioid maintenance treatment for heroin addiction. Standard im analgesic doses are 0.3 mg. Significantly higher doses of sl buprenorphine (up to 24 mg) are necessary to reduce heroin abuse and improve patient retention in opioid addiction treatment. Higher sl doses are used because of the lower bioavailability (approx

35%) of this route of drug administration. Flattened or inverted U-shaped dose-response curves have been demonstrated for physiological and subjective effects of up to 32 mg of sl and up to 16 mg of iv buprenorphine. Even by the iv route, buprenorphine appears to have a ceiling for cardiorespiratory effects and to have a high therapeutic index. It must be cautioned that buprenorphine alone was administered under carefully supervised medical conditions in these studies and that the effects of buprenorphine in combination with other CNS sedatives may produce considerable toxicity. Buprenorphine produces positive subjective responses, indicating a potential for abuse, but the abuse potential does not appear to increase with increasing doses of buprenorphine. The use of a combined buprenorphine-naloxone sl formulation may further reduce its abuse potential.

REFERENCES

1. Lewis JW, Readhead MJ. Novel analgestics and molecular rearrangements in the morphine-thebaine group. XVIII. 3-deoxy-6,14-endo-etheno-6,7,8,14-tetrahydro-oripavines. J Med Chem 1970;13:525-7.
2. Jasinski DR, Pevnick JS, Griffith JD. Human pharmacology and abuse potential of the analgesic buprenorphine. Arch. Gen. Psychiatry 1978;35:501–16.
3. McQuay HJ, Moore RA, Bullingham RES. Buprenorphine kinetics. In: Advances in pain research and therapy, Foley KM, Inturrisi CE eds., New York: Raven, 1986.
4. Iribarne C, Picart D, Dreano Y, Bail JP, Berthou F. Involvement of cytochrome P450 3A4 in n-dealkylation of buprenorphine in human liver microsomes. Life Sci 1997;60(22):1953–64.
5. Payne R. Novel routes of opioid administration: part 1-sublingual and buccal. Primary Care Cancer 1989; January:55–6.
6. Bullingham RES, Dwyer D, Allen MC, Moore RA, McQuay HJ. Sublingual buprenorphine used postoperatively: clinical observations and preliminary pharmacokinetic analysis. Br J Clin Pharmacol 1981;12:117–22.
7. Bullingham RES, McQuay HJ, Porter EJB, Allen MC, Moore RA. Sublingual buprenorphine used postoperatively: ten hour plasma drug concentration analysis. Br J Clin Pharmacol 1982;13:665–73.
8. Weinberg DS, Inturrisi CE, Reidenberg B, Moulin DE, Nip TJ, Wallenstein S, Houde RW, Foley KM. Sublingual absorption of selected opioid analgesics. Clin Pharmacol Ther 1988;44:335–42.
9. Cone EJ, Dickerson SL, Darwin WD, Fudala P, Johnson RE. Elevated drug saliva levels suggest a "depot-like" effect in subjects treated with sublingual buprenorphine. NIDA Res Monogr 1991;105:569.
10. Walter DS, Inturrisi CE. Absorption, distribution, metabolism, and excretion of buprenorphine in animals and humans. In: Buprenorphine: combatting drug abuse with a unique opioid, Cowan A, Lewis JW, eds., New York: Wiley-Liss, 1995.
11. Kuhlman JJ, Levine B, Johnson RE, Fudala PJ, Cone EJ. Relationship of plasma buprenorphine and norbuprenorphine to withdrawal symptoms during dose induc-

tion, maintenance and withdrawal from sublingual buprenorphine. Addiction 1998;93(4):549–59.
12. Cowan A, Doxey JC, Harry EJR. The animal pharmacology of buprenorphine, an oripavine analgesic agent. Br J Pharmac 1977;60:547–54.
13. Wilding IR, Davis SS, Rimoy GH, Rubin P, Kurihara-Bergstrom T, Tipnis V, Berner B, Nightingale J. Pharmacokinetic evaluation of transdermal buprenorphine in man. Intl J Pharmac 1996;132:81–7.
14. Stinchcomb AL, Paliwal A, Dua R, Imoto H, Woodard RW, Flynn GL. Permeation of buprenorphine and its 3-alkyl-ester prodrugs through human skin. Pharm Res 1996;13:1519–23.
15. Fudala PJ, Jaffe JH, Dax EM, Johnson RE. Use of buprenorphine in the treatment of opioid addiction. II. Physiologic and behavioral effects of daily and alternate-day administration and abrupt withdrawal. Clin Pharmacol Ther 1990;47:525–34.
16. Mendelson J, Jones RT, Upton R, and Lin E. Dose-proportionality of sublingual buprenorphine and naloxone tablets. Clin Pharmacol Ther 1998;63(2):204.
17. Mendelson J, Upton R, Lin E, Welm S, Jones RT. Dose proportionality of 4, 8, 16 and 32 mg sublingual buprenorphine solutions. Am Soc Clin Pharmacol Ther 1999;154.
18. Nath RP, Upton RA, Everhart T, Cheung P, Shwonek P, Jones RT, Mendelson JE. Buprenorphine pharmacokinetics: relative bioavailability of sublingual tablet and liquid formulations. J Clin Pharmacol 1999;39:619–23.
19. Mendelson J, Upton R, Jones RT, Jacob P III. Buprenorphine pharmacokinetics: bioequivalence of an 8 mg sublingual tablet formulation. College on Problems of Drug Dependence, Scottsdale, AZ 1998.
20. Wallenstein SL, Kaiko RF, Rogers AG, Houde RW. Clinical analgesic assay of sublingual buprenorphine and intramuscular morphine. In: NIDA research monograph, Harris, L ed. Rockville, MD: NIDA Research Monograph, 1982.
21. de Klerk G, Matti, H, Spierdijk J. Comparative study on the ciculatory and respiratory effects of buprenorphine and methadone. Acta Anaesthesiol Belgica 1981; 32:131–9.
22. Johnson RE, Jaffe JH, Fudala PJ. A controlled trial of buprenorphine treatment for opioid dependence. JAMA 1992;267:2750–55.
23. Kosten TR, Schottenfeld R, Ziedonis D, Falcioni J, Buprenorphine versus methadone maintenance for opioid dependence. J Nerv Ment Dis 1993;181(6):358–64.
24. Ling W, Wesson DR, Charuvastra C, Klett CJ. A controlled trial comparing buprenorphine and methadone maintenance in opioid dependence. Arch Gen Psychiatry 1996;53:401–7.
25. Walsh SL, Preston KL, Stitzer ML, Cone EJ, Bigelow GE. Clinical pharmacology of buprenorphine: ceiling effects at high doses. Clin Pharmacol Ther 1994; 55:569–80.
26. Pickworth WB, Johnson RE, Holicky BA, Cone EJ. Subjective and physiologic effects of intravenous buprenorphine in humans. Clin Pharmacol Ther 1993; 53:570–6.
27. Mello NK, Mendelson JH. Buprenorphine treatment of cocaine and heroin abuse. In: Buprenorphine: combatting drug abuse with a unique opioid. Cowan A, Lewis JW eds. New York: Wiley-Liss, 1995.

28. Preston KL, Silverman K, Umbricht A, DeJesus A, Montoya ID, Schuster CR. Improvement in naltrexone treatment compliance with contingency management. Drug Alcohol Depend 1999;54:127–35.
29. Jasinski DR, Fudala PJ, Johnson RE. Sublingual versus subcutaneous buprenorphine in opiate abusers. Clin Pharmacol Ther 1989;45:513–9.
30. Quigley AJ, Bredemeyer DE, Seow SS. A case of buprenorphine abuse. MJA 1984;142:425–6.
31. Lewis JW. Buprenorphine. Drug Alcohol Depend 1985;14:363–72.
32. Tebbett IR. Analysis of buprenorphine by high-performance liquid chromatography. J Chromatogr 1985;347:411–3.
33. Vanacker B, Vandermeersch E, Tomassen J. Comparison of intramuscular buprenorphine and a buprenorphine/naloxone combination in the treatment of postoperative pain. Curr Med Res Opin 1986;10:139–44.
34. Preston KL, Bigelow GE, Liebson IA. Buprenorphine and naloxone alone and in combination in opioid-dependent humans. Psychopharmacology 1988;94:484–90.
35. Weinhold LL, Preston KL, Farre M, Liebson IA, Bigelow GE. Buprenorphine alone and in combination with naloxone in non-dependent humans. Drug Alcohol Depend 1992;30:263–74.
36. Baster TJ, Gibbs JM, Richardson T. Effect of buprenorphine on the ventilatory response to carbon dioxide. Anaesth Intensive Care 1977;5:128–33.
37. Bickel WK, Stitzer ML, Bigelow GE, Liebson IA, Jasinski DR, Johnson RE. Buprenorphine: dose-related blockade of opioid challenge effects in opioid dependent humans. J Pharmacol Exp Ther 1988;247:47–53.
38. Banks CD. Overdosage of buprenorphine: case report. N Z Med J 1979;89:255–7.
39. Heel RC, Brogden RN, Speight TM, Avery GS. Buprenorphine: A review of its pharmacological properties and therapeutic efficacy. Drugs 1979;17:81–110.
40. McQuay HJ, Bullingham RES, Paterson GMC, Moore RA. Clinical effects of buprenorphine during and after operation. Br J Anaesth 1980;52:1013–9.
41. Teoh SK, Mendelson JH, Mello NK, Kuehnle J, Sintavanarong P, Rhoades EM. Acute interactions of buprenorphine with intravenous cocaine and morphine: an investigational new drug phase I safety evaluation. J Clin Pharmacol 1993;13:87–99.
42. Budd K. High dose buprenorphine for postperative analgesia. Anaesthesia 1981;36:900–3.
43. Faroqui MH, Cole M, Curran J. Buprenorphine, benzodiazepines and respiratory depression. Anaesthesia 1983;38:1002–3.
44. Schmidt JF, Chraemmer-Jorgensen B, Pedersen JE, Risbo A. Postoperative pain relief with naloxone: Severe respiratory depression and pain after high dose buprenorphine. Anaesthesia 1985;40:583–6.
45. Sekar M, Mimpriss TJ. Buprenorphine, benzodiazepines and prolonged respiratory depression. Anaesthesia 1987;42:567–8.
46. Gaulier JM, Marquet P, Lacassie E, Dupuy JL Lachatre G. Fatal intoxication following self-administration of a massive dose of buprenorphine. J Forensic Sci 2000; 45(1):226–8.
47. Zanette G, Manani G, Giusti F, Pittoni G, Ori C. Respiratory depression following administration of low dose buprenorphine as postoperative analgesic after fentanyl balanced anaesthesia. Paediatr Anaesth 1996;6:419–22.

48. Lober C. Buprenorphine. Drug Information Update: Hartford Hosp 1988; 52(5): 285–7.
49. Seyer D, Dif C, Balthazard G, Sciortino V. Traitement de substitution par buprenorphine-haut-dosage: les recommendations sont-elles suivies? Therapie 1998;53:349–54.
50. Ibrahim RB, Wilson JG, Thorsby ME, Edwards DJ. Effect of buprenorphine on CYP3A activity in rat and human liver microsomes. Life Sci 2000;66:1293–8.
51. Saarialho-Kere U, Mattila MJ, Paloheimo M, Seppala T. Psychomotor, respiratory and neuroendocrinological effects of buprenorphine and amitriptyline in healthy volunteers. Eur J Clin Pharmacol 1987;33:139–46.
52. Iribarne C, Picart D, Dreano Y, Berthou F. In vitro interactions between fluoxetine or fluvoxamine and methadone or buprenorphine. Fundam Clin Pharmacol 1998;12:194–9.
53. Iribarne C, Bethou F, Carlhant D, Dreano Y, Picart D, Lohezic F, Riche C. Inhibition of methadone and buprenorphine n-dealkylations by three HIV-1 protease inhibitors. Drug Metab Dispos 1998;26(3):257–60.
54. Hand CW, Baldwin D, Moore RA, Allen MC, McQuay HJ. Radioimmunoassay of buprenorphine with iodine label: analysis of buprenorphine and metabolites in human plasma. Ann Clin Biochem 1986;23:47–53.
55. Ohtani M, Kotaki H, Nishitateno K, Sawada Y, Iga T. Kinetics of respiratory depression in rats induced by buprenorphine and its metabolite, norbuprenorphine. J Pharmacol Exp Ther 1997;281:428–33.
56. Umbricht A, Huestis MA, Cone EJ, Preston KL. Safety of burprenorphine: ceiling for cardio-respiratory effects at high IV doses. NIDA Res Monograph 1998;179:225.
57. Mendelson J, Upton RA, Everhart ET, Jacob P III, Jones RT. Bioavailability of sublingual buprenorphine. J Clin Pharmacol 1997;37(1):31–7.

Chapter 3

High-Dose Buprenorphine for Treatment of Opioid Dependence

Eric C. Strain

1. INTRODUCTION

Buprenorphine was first approved and marketed as an analgesic. When used for this indication, it is typically administered by injection, and the recommended dose is 0.3 mg every 6 h. Higher doses, such as 0.6 mg every 6 h, may be indicated in cases of severe pain. Thus, the recommended total daily analgesic dose is 1.2–2.4 mg.

Early clinical, inpatient laboratory studies that relate to the development of buprenorphine for the treatment of opioid dependence also used parenteral doses of buprenorphine (e.g., see refs. *1* and *2*). However, these studies tested the effects of doses higher than those used for pain control. For example, in a study conducted by Mello and Mendelson *(2)*, subjects were maintained on doses of up to 8 mg/d of subcutaneous (sc) buprenorphine.

These laboratory studies of buprenorphine allowed high-dose administration under the controlled and supervised conditions of an inpatient experimental research unit. However, testing of buprenorphine for the outpatient treatment of opioid dependence meant delivery could no longer be reasonably administered by daily injections, and control of the subject population was diminished (because patients would leave the clinic after dosing). Since buprenorphine has poor oral bioavailability, outpatient clinical trials of buprenorphine for the treatment of opioid dependence have used a sublingual (sl) route of administration. Dosing in early outpatient clinical trials also tended to be low. For example, an early double-blind study comparing sl buprenorphine to oral methadone used daily doses of 2 mg of buprenorphine *(3)* a dose similar to that used for analgesic purposes.

From *Forensic Science and Medicine: Buprenorphine Therapy of Opiate Addiction*
Edited by: P. Kintz and P. Marquet © Humana Press Inc., Totowa, NJ

Subsequent outpatient clinic trials tested increasingly higher doses of buprenorphine (reviewed in more detail later). The use of higher doses of buprenorphine can be understood in light of two pharmacological features of this medication. First is the relatively poor bioavailability of buprenorphine when taken sublingually, compared to parenteral administration *(4)*. While there can be considerable variability among subjects, alcohol solutions of buprenorphine taken sublingually generally deliver about 50% of the dose. The second reason relates to buprenorphine's dose-response curve. Buprenorphine is a mixed agonist-antagonist (a μ partial agonist and a κ antagonist). Preclinical studies have shown that buprenorphine has a bell-shaped dose-response curve with a relatively moderate maximal effect *(5–8)*. This profile suggests that higher doses of buprenorphine could be safely administered to patients without the risks associated with higher doses of full agonist opioids (for example, respiratory depression).

The term *high-dose buprenorphine* can thus be best understood as a comparison of doses used for the treatment of pain and early doses used in the treatment of opioid dependence. Over the course of more than 20 yr of clinical studies with buprenorphine, the tendency is for increasingly higher doses to be used. However, referring to such doses as "high" or "low" is a matter of relative comparison.

A final point regarding the use of the term *high-dose buprenorphine* should be noted. Referring to a dose as low or high can suggest that the dose is ineffective (low) or excessive (high). In this respect, referring to high and low doses should be avoided. In the treatment of opioid dependence, what is necessary is the *effective dose*—the dose that produces the best outcomes for the patient, with minimal adverse effects. This chapter provides a review of the efficacy and safety of buprenorphine when used for the treatment of opioid dependence.

2. BUPRENORPHINE SOLUTION VS TABLETS

Before reviewing studies that have tested the efficacy and safety of buprenorphine for the treatment of opioid dependence, it is important to clarify that studies have differed in the sl form of buprenorphine used. Many early outpatient clinical trials used an sl solution of buprenorphine. Since there are drawbacks to marketing an sl solution, a sublingual tablet form of buprenorphine was then developed. Buprenorphine tablets do not provide a dose equivalent to the solution. While there can be considerable variability among patients, studies have shown that tablets deliver less buprenorphine than a comparable dose in solution *(9,10)*, and one study has quantified this as

50% less *(9)*. When reviewing results from clinical trials, it is important to note the form of delivery (solution vs tablet), especially when drawing cross-study conclusions about dose efficacy.

The remainder of this chapter provides a review of the clinical trials that have tested the efficacy of buprenorphine. The next section reviews results from studies comparing buprenorphine to placebo and the following section reviews clinical trials comparing the efficacy of buprenorphine with that of other medications (primarily methadone). A brief section then addresses the safety and side effects of buprenorphine.

3. EFFICACY OF BUPRENORPHINE VS PLACEBO: CLINICAL TRIALS (TABLE 1)

There have been few placebo-controlled studies of buprenorphine. This relates to both experimental design issues, and concerns about treating opioid-dependent patients with placebo. Each of these points is briefly addressed here.

Designing a placebo-controlled study of opioid dependence treatment can be difficult because of problems associated with maintaining the study blind. Opioid-dependent patients assigned to a placebo condition would quickly determine their condition assignment, either through lack of suppression of spontaneous withdrawal or by an absence of subjective effects produced by the study medication. Unlike studies for most other psychoactive substances, such as antidepressants, both patients and staff could quickly guess the condition assignment for each patient.

Since there are known to be effective treatments for opioid dependence (e.g., methadone, levomethadyl acetate [LAAM]), treating opioid-dependent patients with placebo also can be questioned. Interestingly, in the United States, methadone did not undergo typical placebo-controlled testing for efficacy prior to its approval for the treatment of opioid dependence, although subsequent studies have provided assessments of methadone relative to placebo *(11,12)*. These studies addressed the design problem discussed previously by having some patients undergo a double-blind methadone withdrawal before treatment with placebo. Such a procedure—methadone withdrawal—is not inconsistent with clinical practice and shows how novel designs can be used to address the difficulties in conducting placebo-controlled studies in opioid-dependent patients.

Given these limitations to the design and execution of placebo-controlled studies for the pharmacological treatment of opioid dependence, it is perhaps not surprising that there have been only three such studies testing the efficacy of buprenorphine (Table 1).

Table 1
Placebo-Controlled Studies of Buprenorphine
for Treatment of Opioid Dependence[a]

Reference	No. of patients	Study duration	Buprenorphine Form[b]	Doses[c]	Outcomes
13, Johnson et al., 1995 (DB)	150	14 d	Solution	0, 2, 8 mg	Buprenorphine (regardless of dose) superior to placebo
14, Ling et al., 1998 (DB)	736	16 wk	Solution	1, 4, 8, 16 mg	Buprenorphine (8 mg) superior to placebo (1 mg of buprenorphine)
15, Fudala et al., 1998 (DB)	326	4 wk	Tablet	0, 16, 16/4 mg	Both buprenorphine conditions superior to placebo

[a]DB in the reference column indicates that dosing was double blind.
[b]All studies administered buprenorphine sublingually.
[c]In the Fudala et al. (15) study, doses were placebo (0 mg), buprenorphine alone (16 mg), and buprenorphine (16 mg) combined with naloxone (4 mg); this last condition is indicated by 16/4.

The first study, by Johnson et al. *(13)*, compared three conditions: 0, 2, and 8 mg of daily sl buprenorphine solution. This study utilized a novel, fast-track admission procedure for patients applying to a treatment/research clinic. Applicants would normally have a delay between the time of application and admission, as assessments were completed and eligibility was determined. In this study, special resources were devoted to bringing applicants quickly into the clinic, and avoiding this delay. Thus, time spent on a waiting list for admission was markedly decreased. Study dosing occurred for only 2 wk before all subjects were stabilized on 8 mg/d of sl buprenorphine solution.

Participants ($n = 150$) knew they might receive one of the three doses. After stabilization for 5 d, they could choose to have a double-blind switch to one of the other two conditions (which would be randomly chosen). It was expected that patients initially assigned to placebo ($n = 60$) would request the most switches, those initially assigned to the 2 mg condition ($n=60$) a moderate number of switches, and those initially in the 8-mg group ($n = 30$) the fewest switches.

The results showed that patients on buprenorphine remained on their dose a longer period of time, compared with patients on placebo. Patients on buprenorphine also used less illicit opioids, as determined by urine testing. This effect on urine results was primarily seen in the 72 male patients, but not in the 31 female patients who completed the study. This sex difference may reflect the lower number of female patients. Finally, there were no marked differences between the 2- and 8-mg conditions. This may reflect the relatively short duration of the study period.

The second clinical trial, by Ling et al. *(14)*, testing the efficacy of buprenorphine compared to placebo, was a multisite study conducted in the 1990s in the United States. Dosing in this study was double blind, and patients ($n = 736$) were randomly assigned to either 1, 4, 8, or 16 mg of daily sl buprenorphine solution. The 1-mg dose of buprenorphine used was selected to serve as a placebo condition, and the primary planned comparison was between the 8- and 1-mg groups.

Results from this study showed that 8 mg was superior to 1 mg on a variety of outcome measures such as treatment retention, mean percentage of opioid-negative urine samples, percentage of patients with 13 consecutive opioid-negative urine samples (i.e., 1 mo of abstinence), and mean number of opioid-negative urines. Secondary outcome measures, such as self-reported global ratings of the severity of drug problems, also showed significant differences between the 1- and 8-mg groups. Furthermore, while the primary study question was whether 8 mg of buprenorphine was superior to placebo (1 mg), the inclusion of the 4- and 16-mg conditions allowed assessment of these conditions as well. A dose effect was seen across the four doses tested, with the best outcomes in the 16-mg condition.

The final study, by Fudala et al. *(15)*, still had not been published in the peer-reviewed literature as of February 2001, but it is available in abstract form after presentation at a scientific conference. This was a multisite study comparing buprenorphine alone (16 mg), buprenorphine combined with naloxone (16/4 mg), and placebo. Unlike the previous two studies, this study used a tablet form of buprenorphine, so the effective dose delivered is not unlike the 8-mg dose conditions in the two other placebo-controlled studies (since the other two studies used buprenorphine solution). Participants who completed the 4-wk study phase were eligible to then enter a 48-wk open-label dosing study.

The notable feature to this study's outcome is that an interim analysis of results led to the decision to stop the study early because outcomes for the two buprenorphine conditions were so clearly better than for placebo. Quantitative results were not published in the abstract, but both buprenorphine conditions were significantly better than placebo on outcomes of urine samples tested for illicit opioids, as well as measures of opioid craving and global impression ratings.

3.1. Summary of Placebo-Controlled Studies

While there have only been three studies comparing buprenorphine to placebo, all three enrolled substantial numbers of patients, used good clinical trial designs (e.g., double-blind dosing, random assignment to conditions, objective measures of drug use), and found similar results. In addition, all three studies attempted to address the difficulties in conducting placebo-controlled studies in opioid-dependent patients. Given the convergence of results from the three studies, it seems unlikely that there would need to be further placebo-controlled studies of buprenorphine for the treatment of opioid dependence.

4. Efficacy of Buprenorphine vs Other Medications: Clinical Trials (Tables 2 and 3)

There have been numerous reports on the outpatient clinical use of buprenorphine for the treatment of opioid dependence (e.g., see refs. *16–19*), and these studies provide valuable information about clinical experience and outcomes associated with the use of buprenorphine for the treatment of opioid dependence. However, for purposes of this review, only studies that included a control medication, were published in English, and utilized a period of stable

Table 2
Studies of Buprenorphine vs Other Medications for the Treatment of Opioid Dependence[a]

Reference	No. of subjects	Study duration (wk)	Buprenorphine Form[b]	Buprenorphine Dose(s)	Comparison medication, dose	Outcomes Retention	Outcomes Opioid urinalysis
3, Bickel et al., 1988 (DB)	45	13	Solution	2 mg	M30 mg	B = M	B = M
21, Johnson et al., 1992 (DB)	162	17	Solution	8 mg	M20 + M60 mg	B > M20	B, M60 > M20
22, Kosten et al., 1993 (DB)	125	24	Solution	2 + 6 mg	M35 + M65 mg	M > B	M > B
23, Strain et al., 1994 (DB)	51	26	Solution	8–16 mg	M50–90 mg	B = M	B = M
24, Strain et al., 1994 (DB)	164	26	Solution	8–16 mg	M50–90 mg	B = M	B = M
25, Ling et al., 1996 (DB)	225	52	Solution	8 mg	M30 + M80 mg	M80 > B, M30	M80 > B, M30
26, Schottenfeld et al., 1997 (DB)	116	24	Solution	4 + 12 mg	M20 + M65 mg	No difference between groups	B12, M65 > B4, M20
27, Oliveto et al., 1999 (DB)	180	13	Solution	12 mg	M65 mg	B = M	M > B
28, Fischer et al., 1999	60	24	Tablet	2–8 mg	Up to M80 mg	M > B	B > M
29, Pani et al., 2000 (DB)	72	26	Tablet	8 mg	M60 mg	M > B (trend)	B = M
30, Mattick et al., 1999 (DB)	405	13	Tablet	up to 32 mg	M up to 150 mg	B = M	B = M
31, Johnson et al., 2000 (DB)	220	17	Solution	16–32 mg 3X/wk	LAAM 75–115 mg 3X/wk, M20 + M60–100 mg	B, LAAM, M60–100 > M20	B, LAAM, M60–100 > M20
32, Petitjean et al., 2001 (DB)	58	6	Tablet	4–16 mg	M30–120 mg	M > B	B = M

[a]DB in the reference column indicates that dosing was double-blind, and references without DB were open label; B, buprenorphine; M, methadone.
[b]All studies administered buprenorphine sublingually.

Table 3
Studies of Buprenorphine vs Methadone in Overall Rates (%) of Opioid-Positive Urine Samples[a]

Reference	Methadone dose (mg)					Buprenorphine dose (mg)[b]			
	20	30–35	54–60	65–67	≥70	4	8–12	16–18	22–24
21, Johnson et al., 1992	71		56					47	
22, Kosten et al., 1993		48		49		73	76		
23, Strain et al., 1994				60					55
24, Strain et al., 1994			47					55	
25, Ling et al., 1996		55			38			55	
26, Schottenfeld et al., 1997	72			45			77		58
29, Pani et al., 2000			34				40		
32, Petitjean et al., 2001					60		62		

[a]Comparable overall rates of opioid-positive urine samples were not available for the following studies: Bickel et al. (3), Oliveto et al. (27), Mattick et al. (30), Johnson et al. (31).
[b]Doses shown are for the tablet form of buprenorphine and are daily doses. Doses of buprenorphine that were originally delivered as solution were doubled to give an approximately equivalent dose in the tablet form.

dosing (i.e., did not have the primary purpose of determining efficacy of buprenorphine as a withdrawal agent) are included. Virtually all these studies compared buprenorphine to methadone (with the exception of one clinical trial), and until 1999, all reports used the solution form of buprenorphine. While an exhaustive review of these studies is beyond the scope of this chapter, the highlights of each study are briefly summarized. A review of the clinical use of buprenorphine for the treatment of opioid dependence was published in 1995 *(20)*, and a special supplement on buprenorphine's use in the treatment of opioid dependence is due to be published in the journal *Drug and Alcohol Dependence*.

An early controlled, outpatient clinical trial comparing buprenorphine to methadone was published in 1988 *(3)*. The study compared 2 mg of buprenorphine solution ($n = 22$) to 30 mg of daily methadone ($n = 23$); while the total study duration was 13 wk, stable dosing occurred for only the first 3 wk. Participants then underwent a withdrawal between wk 4 and 7 and received placebo dosing between wk 8 and 13. A unique feature of this study was the inclusion of a 6-mg intramuscular (im) hydromorphone challenge during the second week of treatment. Hydromorphone is a prototypic µ agonist opioid, and response to the challenge provided an assessment of the blockade efficacy of buprenorphine and methadone.

The results showed that buprenorphine and methadone were similar on outcomes of treatment retention and opioid-positive urinalyses (which were collected and tested three to four times per week). However, methadone was significantly more effective in attenuating the effects of the hydromorphone challenge, as assessed by the physiological measure pupil diameter and subjective measures. This study demonstrated that buprenorphine could be used in the outpatient treatment of opioid dependence but suggests that the dose used (2 mg/d) was too low. In addition, the study had a short duration of maintenance dosing, and outcomes were poor once dose reductions began for both medications.

The next clinical trial, by Johnson et al. *(21)*, can be seen as building on the Bickel et al. *(3)* study, with several differences in the study design. It enrolled a larger number of subjects (53 participants on buprenorphine, 55 on 20 mg of daily methadone, and 54 on 60 mg of daily methadone), tested a higher dose of buprenorphine (8 mg/d), and had a longer duration (17 wk of induction/stabilization). The inclusion of the lower dose of methadone provided a control condition and the added value of an assessment of the dose-related efficacy of methadone. Urine samples were collected and tested three times per week, and participants were offered but not required to attend counseling services.

Patients assigned to the buprenorphine condition had significantly better retention than those patients in the 20-mg methadone condition, whereas there was no significant difference between the two methadone groups for treatment retention. Although not significant, there was slightly better retention at the end of 17 wk for the buprenorphine group (42%) vs the 60-mg methadone group (32%). Both patients on buprenorphine and 60 mg of methadone also had significantly lower rates of opioid-positive urine samples (47 and 56%, respectively) compared with patients on 20 mg of methadone (71%) (Table 3). Among the subset of patients who completed the 17-wk phase of the study, patients on buprenorphine had significantly lower rates of opioid-positive urine samples (41%) vs both 60 and 20 mg of methadone (57 and 61%, respectively). Thus, this study showed that 8 mg of daily sl buprenorphine produced outcomes comparable to 60 mg of methadone, with some suggestion that this dose of buprenorphine might even have better outcomes than 60 mg of methadone.

These first two clinical trials were both conducted in Baltimore, MD (the Bickel et al. *[3]* study at Johns Hopkins University, and the Johnson et al. *[21]* study at the National Institute on Drug Abuse Intramural Research Program). In 1993, a study from Yale University (New Haven, CT), by Kosten et al. *(22)*, comparing two doses of buprenorphine and two doses of methadone was published. This study randomly assigned subjects to either 35 or 65 mg of methadone (34 and 35 subjects, respectively), or 2 or 6 mg of buprenorphine (28 subjects in each group). Notably, in the Johnson et al. *(21)* study, patients were instructed to hold sl solution under the tongue for at least 10 min, while in the Kosten et al. *(22)* study patients were instructed to hold the solution under the tongue for at least 2 min. Urine samples were collected and tested once per week in the present study.

Analyses of the results showed that treatment retention was significantly better for the methadone groups vs the buprenorphine groups, but there was no significant difference between the low- and high-dose groups within each medication type for treatment retention. Urinalysis results also showed the methadone groups to have better outcomes than the buprenorphine groups. The overall rate of opioid-positive urine samples was 49 and 48% for the 65- and 35-mg methadone conditions, respectively, while it was 76 and 73% for the 6- and 2-mg buprenorphine conditions, respectively (Table 3). This study's results, which show methadone superior to buprenorphine, should be interpreted with two cautionary notes. First, the duration buprenorphine was held under the tongue might have been too short, so patients in the buprenorphine conditions received doses lower than intended (and not comparable with other studies using these doses). Second, the study did not show a dose effect for methadone—a somewhat surprising finding.

Two studies published in 1994 were conducted by the same research group and used a similar research design, so they are summarized together here. Both studies compared a dose range of buprenorphine with a dose range of methadone using a flexible dosing procedure. Studies that test fixed doses of buprenorphine and methadone can show differences in medications that reflect noncomparable doses, rather than true medication differences. For example, a study comparing 8 mg of buprenorphine to 20 mg of methadone would probably find buprenorphine to be superior, while another study comparing 2 mg of buprenorphine to 100 mg of methadone would probably show methadone as superior—but outcomes would reflect dose differences, not necessarily medication differences. The present pair of studies compared 8–16 mg of buprenorphine to 50–90 mg of methadone, in an effort to address this methodological shortcoming. Participants were treated for 16 wk, and urine samples were collected and tested three times per week. The primary difference between the studies was the sample sizes and the target drug use. One study *(24)* enrolled a total of 164 subjects (84 treated with buprenorphine and 80 with methadone) and delivered double-blind dose increases if there was evidence of continued illicit opioid use. The other study *(23)* enrolled 51 patients (24 treated with buprenorphine and 27 with methadone) and provided dose increases if there was evidence of either illicit opioid or cocaine use. Subjects in both studies were instructed to hold the sl solution under the tongue for at least 5 min (and were timed by nursing staff).

Results from both studies were similar. There was no significant difference in treatment retention for patients treated with buprenorphine or methadone, and rates of opioid-positive urine samples were not significantly different for the two medications. The average dose of buprenorphine used in the larger study *(24)* was 8.9 mg/d, and the average dose of methadone was 54 mg. This suggests that the Johnson et al. *(21)* and Kosten et al. *(22)* studies used buprenorphine doses that were too low relative to the higher dose methadone conditions in those studies. In the present study of 164 patients, the rate of opioid-positive urine samples for patients treated with methadone was 47%, similar to the rates found in the Johnson et al. *(21)* (60-mg group: 56%) and Kosten et al. *(22)* (65-mg group: 49%) methadone groups (Table 3). Finally, it should be noted that there was no evidence from the smaller of the present studies *(23)* that buprenorphine or methadone produced selective attenuation of cocaine use.

The next outpatient clinical trial comparing buprenorphine to methadone tested higher daily doses of methadone (30 and 80 mg) but used what was becoming a standard test dose of buprenorphine (8 mg of solution) over a longer period of time than any previous study—1 yr *(25)*. This was also the largest study conducted up to that time, with 75 patients in each of the three dose conditions. Notably, patients were instructed to hold the sl solution under the tongue for up to 5 min. Urine samples were collected and tested three times per week, and primary outcome analyses focused on the first 26 wk of the study (and used the 1 yr data for safety assessments).

Results from the first 26 wk of this study showed that patients in the 80-mg methadone group had better retention than both the 30-mg methadone and the buprenorphine groups, but there was no significant difference in retention for the 30-mg methadone and buprenorphine groups. Assessment of opioid use, based on urinalysis testing over the 26-wk period, also showed that the higher methadone group had significantly better outcome than the other two conditions (38% opioid-positive urine samples), with no significant difference between buprenorphine and the lower-dose methadone condition (both 55% opioid-positive urine samples; Table 3). In retrospect, the superior outcomes for the 80-mg methadone condition are perhaps not unexpected, since 8 mg of daily sl buprenorphine is equivalent to 50–60 mg of daily methadone. However, the somewhat surprising result from this study is that 8 mg of buprenorphine was not superior to 30 mg of methadone. A review of the reported results does not show even a suggestion of a difference between 8 mg of buprenorphine and 30 mg of methadone. These outcomes suggested that estimates of buprenorphine's efficacy relative to methadone might be overly optimistic.

In 1997, a report on a study of buprenorphine vs methadone in the treatment of opioid-dependent patients with concurrent cocaine abuse or dependence was published *(26)*. The study had four treatment groups: 4 mg of buprenorphine ($n = 29$), 12 mg of buprenorphine ($n = 30$), 20 mg of methadone ($n = 30$), and 65 mg of methadone ($n = 28$). Urine samples were collected either twice or thrice weekly. A primary aim of the study was to determine whether buprenorphine was superior to methadone in the treatment of cocaine abuse in this population of patients.

Interestingly, there was no significant difference among the four groups for treatment retention. However, there were significant differences on rates of opioid-positive urine samples: both high-dose conditions had lower rates of opioid-positive urines when compared with the two low-dose conditions. There was no significant difference between the 12-mg buprenorphine and 65-mg methadone conditions, or between the 4-mg buprenorphine and 20-mg methadone conditions. The overall rate of opioid-positive urine samples for the 65-mg condition was 45%, and the rate of opioid-positive urine samples for the 12-mg buprenorphine condition was 58% (Table 3). Finally, one of the primary purposes of the study was to determine whether there was differential efficacy of buprenorphine vs methadone on cocaine use; no such effect was found.

The next study reviewed here also enrolled opioid-dependent patients with concurrent regular cocaine use (27). The primary purpose of the study was to test the efficacy of desipramine vs placebo in the treatment of cocaine abuse, but the study design provides an indirect assessment of buprenorphine versus methadone efficacy for opioid use (i.e., through a review of outcomes for patients treated with placebo rather than active desipramine). While the total enrollment in the study was 180, only one-half of the patients are relevant to the present review: there were 45 patients treated with buprenorphine (12 mg/d of solution) and placebo and 45 with methadone (65 mg/d) and placebo. Notably, like the Kosten et al. (22) study, participants held the sl solution for 2 min. Participants provided urine samples tested three times per week, and the trial lasted 13 wk.

There was no significant difference in treatment retention (although it is important to point out that the survival analysis for this study included all four conditions, not simply the two of interest to the present review). A graph showing treatment retention over time shows no evidence of a difference between the two groups of interest (buprenorphine and placebo vs methadone and placebo). Results from this study for urinalysis testing were presented in a series of figures, but percentage of urinalyses positive for opioids were not provided. Furthermore, a complicated set of analyses were conducted, since it appeared that there were sex and time differences found for urinalysis outcomes. It appears that there was a mild, but significant effect for methadone to produce better outcomes than buprenorphine. However, these differences may be primarily in men, and associated with a more rapid reduction in illicit opioid use, rather than an overall greater decline once patients were stabilized on each medication.

Fischer et al. (28) conducted a study comparing buprenorphine to methadone in the outpatient treatment of opioid dependence, but it was not a double-blind study. It is included here because it was one of the first comparisons of buprenorphine vs methadone done in Europe, it enrolled a moderately large sample of subjects (30 in each medication condition), and it is the first published comparison that used the tablet form of buprenorphine. Doses were either 2 or 8 mg of daily buprenorphine (the 8-mg dose was given as 4 mg twice daily), or up to 80 mg of daily methadone. Patients were seen and received doses under staff supervision for the first 3 wk of the study, but then were seen every other day and received take-home doses for nonclinic days. Urine samples were collected and tested one to two times per week.

Treatment retention was clearly superior for the patients in the methadone group. By the end of the study, patients who remained on buprenorphine had significantly less illicit opioid use compared with patients who remained on methadone, although this difference was not seen when results were examined using an intent-to-treat analysis. However, these results must be interpreted with two cautionary notes. First, the maximum dose of buprenorphine used (8-mg tablet) is equivalent to about 30 mg of methadone; thus, the study did not use maximum equivalent doses. Second, the open nature of the study means that expectancy effects could influence outcomes. Despite these limitations, this study provides further evidence of buprenorphine's relative efficacy, and the project utilized several nicely employed features of a well-designed and conducted clinical trial.

In 2000, Pani et al. *(29)* conducted a second European-based clinical trial comparing buprenorphine to methadone. This was a multisite, double-blind study that used good clinical trials procedures, and it represents the first published double-blind trial comparing buprenorphine tablets to methadone. It compared daily buprenorphine (8 mg delivered as tablets; $n = 38$) to daily methadone (60 mg; $n = 34$). The study duration was 6 mo, and all dosing was done under supervision each day (i.e., there were no take-home doses of medications). Urine samples were collected and tested weekly.

There was no significant difference between groups for treatment retention, although there was a trend for the methadone patients to have better retention. This may be related to early dropouts, which appeared to be more frequent in the buprenorphine group (primarily in the first week). These retention results raise the question of whether a more rapid dose induction procedure might be needed with buprenorphine tablets. (Buprenorphine doses were increased by 2 mg every other day in this study.) Results from urine testing found no significant difference between buprenorphine and methadone groups—a slightly surprising finding, given the relative inequality of the doses used for comparison since an 8-mg buprenorphine tablet is equivalent to approx 30 mg of methadone.

The next study, by Mattick et al. *(30)*, was conducted in Australia, and has not been published in the peer-reviewed literature, but it has been presented at a scientific conference and was reviewed at a meeting in London (March 2000). It is reviewed here because it represents the largest clinical trial comparing buprenorphine to methadone, it used the tablet form of buprenorphine, and it had a flexible dosing procedure with daily doses of buprenorphine and methadone that were higher than in previous studies. However, many of the methodological features of this study are not available at the present time.

The results showed that the average dose of methadone and buprenorphine was 54 and 10 mg respectively. While these doses are similar to the flexible dosing study results described earlier *(24)*, a tablet form of buprenorphine was used (whereas the Strain et al. *[24]* study used solution). Thus, the present study is not entirely consistent with the earlier study, since in the present study an equivalent dose of buprenorphine solution would be approx 5 mg. In the present study, there was no significant difference between the two groups in treatment retention, although methadone patients did have nonsignificantly better retention. Interestingly, this difference seemed to occur during the induction phase of treatment, like the differences noted in Pani et al. *(29)*. Urine test results for illicit opioids also were not significantly different between the two groups. Patients were transferred from daily buprenorphine dosing to alternate-day dosing; ninety-six percent of patients were successfully transitioned to alternate-day dosing during the course of the study. In summary, this study found that buprenorphine and methadone produced similar outcomes when doses were titrated for each patient, although the average dose of buprenorphine appears to be somewhat low compared to the average dose of methadone.

Also in 2000, results from a large clinical trial that directly compared methadone, buprenorphine, and LAAM were published *(31)*. This is the only large outpatient clinical trial to date that has compared buprenorphine to LAAM. The study provided daily doses of a higher dose of methadone (60–100 mg; $n = 55$), a lower dose of methadone (20 mg; $n = 55$), thrice weekly LAAM (75–115 mg; $n = 55$), and thrice weekly buprenorphine (16–32 mg; $n = 55$). Besides comparing thrice weekly buprenorphine to LAAM, the study employed several other novel features (such as a rescue procedure for patients who were continuing to have illicit opioid use, and flexible dosing procedures).

Treatment retention was significantly better for all three groups compared to the lower-dose methadone group, but there was no significant difference between buprenorphine and LAAM, or buprenorphine and higher-dose methadone for treatment retention. Similarly, there was an overall significant effect for illicit opioid use as measured by urine testing, with the best outcomes associated with LAAM, similar rates of use for buprenorphine and the higher-dose methadone group, and the poorest outcomes for the lower-dose methadone group. Thus, this study showed that thrice weekly buprenorphine, delivered as a solution and given under a flexible dosing procedure, could produce outcomes similar to doses of 60–100 mg of daily methadone. In addition, thrice-weekly buprenorphine had similar outcomes to thrice weekly LAAM.

The final study that compared buprenorphine to methadone, which was conducted in Switzerland, also used a flexible dosing procedure and employed the tablet form of buprenorphine *(32)*. The daily doses of buprenorphine were between 4 and 16 mg ($n = 27$) and of methadone were between 30 and 120 mg ($n = 31$). Urine samples were collected weekly.

The average daily dose of buprenorphine was 10.5 mg and of methadone was 70 mg. Treatment retention was significantly better for patients in the methadone condition. Attrition for the buprenorphine patients primarily occurred in the first few days of treatment (as has been noted in other studies; e.g., Pani et al. *(29)*; Marrick et al., *(30)*. While retention was better for the methadone group, there was no significant difference between groups in the rate of opioid-positive urine samples (Table 3).

4.1. Summary of Studies Comparing Buprenorphine to Other Medications

Virtually all of the reviewed outpatient clinical trials compared daily buprenorphine to daily methadone. A few points can be concluded from these studies. First, patients treated with buprenorphine often had similar outcomes to those treated with methadone. Second, differences in treatment retention, when found, seemed to occur in the first days of buprenorphine treatment. This suggests that further refinement of the buprenorphine induction procedure may be needed, or that buprenorphine is not as effective in maintaining patients in treatment during the first days of dose stabilization. Third, some studies that found differential efficacy between methadone and buprenorphine had methodological differences that may account for outcomes (such as a short duration of time that buprenorphine solution was held under the tongue). Finally, it is worth noting that no studies used high doses of buprenorphine— while some studies have provided the option in their design *(30)*, most used relatively low doses. There is a logic suggesting that buprenorphine, since it is a partial agonist, may not be as useful for patients with high levels of physical dependence (vs methadone). However, this has not been addressed in a controlled study. Taken together, the studies reviewed here as well as in the previous section provide an impressive body of clinical experience documenting that buprenorphine is more effective than placebo, and that it can achieve outcomes similar to those found with methadone.

5. SAFETY AND SIDE EFFECTS OF BUPRENORPHINE

Several of the clinical trials reviewed included assessments of safety and side effects for buprenorphine. While outcomes for efficacy measures are generally provided in detail, results from these safety assessments are usually relatively brief. In general, buprenorphine is a safe and well-tolerated medication that produces a profile of side effects similar to those seen with metha-

High-Dose Buprenorphine Treatment

done. For example, in both Johnson et al. *(21,31)* studies, as well as the Ling et al. *(25)* and Pani et al. *(29)* studies, no differential pattern for side effects was seen for buprenorphine vs methadone dose conditions.

One report specifically addressed the safety and side effects of buprenorphine when used in the treatment of opioid dependence *(33)*. None of the side effects and adverse events were definitely related to buprenorphine, and of those thought to be probably related, the majority (93%) was constipation (with the other 7% sedation/drowsiness). However, no control condition was employed in these analyses, so these rates and severity cannot be compared, e.g., to methadone.

One other study on adverse events and buprenorphine should be noted *(34)*. This review of patients treated with buprenorphine ($n = 120$) found that patients with a history of hepatitis were more likely to develop increases in liver enzyme tests (aspartate aminotransferase and alanine aminotransferase) compared with buprenorphine-treated patients without a history of hepatitis. The assessment of liver function in outpatients with opioid dependence can be difficult, since other intervening factors can also alter liver function tests (e.g., alcohol use, other drug use). In addition, this study did not include a control condition, such as methadone, so the results should be interpreted with caution. Still, until more studies are available that address the question of how chronic buprenorphine use, hepatitis, and liver function tests may be related, the results from this retrospective report suggest that caution and monitoring of liver function may be warranted in opioid-dependent patients who are to be treated with buprenorphine, and who have a history of hepatitis.

Finally, while not a direct side effect of buprenorphine, it is important to note that several fatalities reported from France appear to be related to the use of buprenorphine with a benzodiazepine *(35,36)*. This interaction is probably similar to other potentially lethal combinations of sedative medications and drugs of abuse (e.g., alcohol and a benzodiazepine). Use of a benzodiazepine in a patient maintained on buprenorphine is probably best avoided.

6. SUMMARY AND CONCLUSIONS

The purpose of this chapter is to review what is known about the efficacy and safety of higher-dose buprenorphine when used for the treatment of opioid dependence. Numerous clinical trials have examined buprenorphine's efficacy, primarily compared to methadone, a few to placebo, and one to LAAM. After reviewing these reports, it can be concluded with confidence that buprenorphine is useful in the treatment of opioid dependence—especially compared to placebo. Buprenorphine is not superior to methadone, and there is a tendency for higher doses of methadone to produce better outcomes than buprenorphine. However, this may simply reflect a less aggressive strategy used for buprenorphine doses in these studies. While current practice probably views "high-dose" buprenorphine as doses of 8–16 mg/d of solution (or 16–32 mg/d of tablets), further clinical experience and controlled studies may find that these are moderate doses and that higher daily doses produce better outcomes for many patients. Buprenorphine appears to be safe, although further examination of its effects among patients with hepatitis appears warranted.

This review did not include other areas of interest associated with the use of buprenorphine for the treatment of opioid dependence. In particular, two topics were not reviewed. The first is the efficacy of less than daily dosing of buprenorphine. Numerous studies have been conducted with less than daily buprenorphine dosing *(37–41)*, and results from these studies demonstrate that buprenorphine can be effectively used on a less than daily basis. While this topic is of interest, the practical need for less than daily dosing will probably vary as a function of the circumstances under which buprenorphine is used. If buprenorphine is provided by physicians as a part of routine office-based practice (e.g., with a monthly prescription), then daily vs alternate-day dosing may have little relevance to most patients. If buprenorphine is provided in clinics (like the current methadone delivery system in the United States), then alternate-day dosing may have distinct advantages. The most important practical point about alternate-day dosing is that doses must be increased to compensate for the longer between-dose time interval.

The second topic is the use of buprenorphine for medically managed withdrawal (or detoxification). Both clinical experience and controlled studies, primarily with the analgesic form of buprenorphine, suggest that buprenorphine can be effective for the treatment of opioid withdrawal *(42–44)*. While medically managed withdrawal using buprenorphine seems to have become common practice in some areas (e.g., inpatient medical wards at some hospitals in the United States), routine treatment of opioid-dependent patients will probably not involve such procedures.

Finally, many of the studies reviewed here have compared buprenorphine to methadone. Such clinical trials represent one aspect of the medicalization of substance abuse treatment and are important both in terms of outcomes and through the demonstration that the substance abuse field can provide controlled assessments similar to other areas of medicine. For much of the world, methadone is the current standard of care for the pharmacological treatment of opioid dependence and, hence, is the logical comparison medication. However, the results from these studies should not be interpreted as showing that one medication is better than the other. Neither is clearly superior, both are effective, and the field of substance abuse treatment is strengthened by the addition of options in the available medications. Like the development of new medications for hypertension, schizophrenia, or diabetes, the development of a new therapeutic option—buprenorphine—for the treatment of opioid dependence is a welcome step that complements the other treatment options currently available.

ACKNOWLEDGMENT

This work was supported by US Public Health Service Scientist Development Award K02 DA00332 from the National Institue on Drug Abuse.

REFERENCES

1. Jasinski DR, Pevnick JS, Griffith JD. Human pharmacology and abuse potential of the analgesic buprenorphine: a potential agent for treating narcotic addiction. Arch Gen Psychiatry 1978;35:501–16.
2. Mello NK, Mendelson JH. Buprenorphine suppresses heroin use by heroin addicts. Science 1980;207:657–9.
3. Bickel WK, Stitzer ML, Bigelow GE, Liebson IA, Jasinski DR, Johnson RE. A clinical trial of buprenorphine: comparison with methadone in the detoxification of heroin addicts. Clin Pharmacol Ther 1988;43:72–8.
4. Kuhlman JJ, Lalani S, Magluilo J, Levine B, Darwin WD. Human pharmacokinetics of intravenous, sublingual, and buccal buprenorphine. J Anal Toxicol 1996; 20:369–78.
5. Cowan A, Doxey JC, Harry EJ. The animal pharmacology of buprenorphine, an oripavine analgesic agent. Br J Pharmacol 1977;60:547–54.
6. Doxey JC, Everitt JE, Frank LW, MacKenzie JE. A comparison of the effects of buprenorphine and morphine on the blood gases of conscious rats. Br J Pharmacol 1982;75:118P.
7. Dum JE, Herz A. In vivo receptor binding of the opiate partial agonist, buprenorphine, correlated with its agonistic and antagonistic actions. Br J Pharmacol 1981;74:627–33.
8. Lizasoain I, Leza JC, Lorenzo P. Buprenorphine: bell-shaped dose-response curve for its antagonist effects. Gen Pharmacol 1991;22:297–300.
9. Nath RP, Upton RA, Everhart ET, Cheung P, Shwonek P, Jones RT, Mendelson JE. Buprenorphine pharmacokinetics: relative bioavailability of sublingual tablet and liquid formulations. J Clin Pharmacol 1999;39:619–23.
10. Schuh KJ, Johanson CE Pharmacokinetic comparison of the buprenorphine sublingual liquid and tablet. Drug Alcohol Depend 1999;56:55–60.
11. Newman RG, Whitehill WB. Double-blind comparison of methadone and placebo maintenance treatments of narcotic addicts in Hong Kong. Lancet 1979;2:485–8.
12. Strain EC, Stitzer ML, Liebson IA, Bigelow GE. Dose-response effects of methadone in the treatment of opioid dependence. Ann Intern Med 1993;119:23–7.
13. Johnson RE, Eissenberg T, Stitzer ML, Strain EC, Liebson IA, Bigelow GE. A placebo controlled clinical trial of buprenorphine as a treatment for opioid dependence. Drug Alcohol Depend 1995;40:17–25.

14. Ling W, Charuvastra C, Collins JF, et al. Buprenorphine maintenance treatment of opiate dependence: a multicenter, randomized clinical trial. Addiction 1998; 93:475–86.
15. Fudala PJ, Bridge TP, Herbert S, Chiang CN, Leiderman DB A multi-site efficacy evaluation of a buprenorphine/naloxone product for opiate dependence treatment. NIDA Res Monogr 1998;179:105.
16. Compton PA, Wesson DR, Charuvastra VC, Ling W. Buprenorphine as a pharmacotherapy for opiate addiction: what dose provides a therapeutic response? Am J Addict 1996;5:220–30.
17. Kosten TR, Morgan C, Kleber HD. Treatment of heroin addicts using buprenorphine. Am J Drug Alcohol Abuse 1991;17:119–28.
18. Reisinger M. Buprenorphine as new treatment for heroin dependence. Drug Alcohol Depend 1985;16:257–62.
19. Seow SS, Quigley AJ, Ilett KF, Dusci LJ, Swensen G, Harrison-Stewart A, Rappeport L. Buprenorphine: a new maintenance opiate? Med J Aust 1986;144:407–11.
20. Bickel WK, Amass L. Buprenorphine treatment of opioid dependence: a review. Exp Clin Psychopharmacol 1995;3:477–89.
21. Johnson RE, Jaffe JH, Fudala PJ. A controlled trial of buprenorphine treatment for opioid dependence. JAMA 1992;267:2750–5.
22. Kosten TR, Schottenfeld R, Ziedonis D, Falcioni J. Buprenorphine versus methadone maintenance for opioid dependence. J Nerv Ment Dis 1993;181:358–64.
23. Strain EC, Stitzer ML, Liebson IA, Bigelow GE. Buprenorphine versus methadone in the treatment of opioid-dependent cocaine users. Psychopharmacology (Berl) 1994;116:401–6.
24. Strain EC, Stitzer ML, Liebson IA, Bigelow GE. Comparison of buprenorphine and methadone in the treatment of opioid dependence. Am J Psychiatry 1994; 151:1025–30.
25. Ling W, Wesson DR, Charuvastra C, Klett CJ. A controlled trial comparing buprenorphine and methadone maintenance in opioid dependence. Arch Gen Psychiatry 1996;53:401–7.
26. Schottenfeld RS, Pakes JR, Oliveto A, Ziedonis D, Kosten TR. Buprenorphine vs methadone maintenance treatment for concurrent opioid dependence and cocaine abuse. Arch Gen Psychiatry 1997;54:713–20.
27. Oliveto AH, Feingold A, Schottenfeld R, Jatlow P, Kosten TR. Desipramine in opioid-dependent cocaine abusers maintained on buprenorphine vs methadone. Arch Gen Psychiatry 1999;56:812–20.
28. Fischer G, Gombas W, Eder H, et al. Buprenorphine versus methadone maintenance for the treatment of opioid dependence. Addiction 1999;94:1337–47.
29. Pani PP, Maremmani I, Pirastu R, Tagliamonte A, Gessa GL. Buprenorphine: a controlled clinical trial in the treatment of opioid dependence. Drug Alcohol Depend 2000;60:39–50.
30. Mattick RP, Ali R, White J, O'Brien S, Wolk S, Danz C. A randomised double-blind trial of buprenorphine tablets versus methadone syrup for maintenance therapy: efficacy and cost-effectiveness. NIDA Res Monogr 1999;180:77.

31. Johnson RE, Chutuape MA, Strain EC, Walsh SL, Stitzer ML, Bigelow GE. A comparison of levomethadyl acetate, buprenorphine, and methadone for opioid dependence. N Engl J Med 2000;343:1290–7.
32. Petitjean S, Stohler R, Deglon J, Livoti S, Waldvogel D, Uehlinger C, Ladewig D. Double-blind randomized trial of buprenorphine and methadone in opiate dependence. Drug Alcohol Depend 2001;62:97–104.
33. Lange WR, Fudala PJ, Dax EM, Johnson RE. Safety and side-effects of buprenorphine in the clinical management of heroin addiction. Drug Alcohol Depend 1990;26:19–28.
34. Petry NM, Bickel WK, Piasecki D, Marsch LA, Badger GJ. Elevated liver enzyme levels in opioid-dependent patients with hepatitis treated with buprenorphine. Am J Addict 2000;9:265–9.
35. Reynaud M, Petit G, Potard D, Courty P. Six deaths linked to concomitant use of buprenorphine and benzodiazepines. Addiction 1998;93:1385–92.
36. Tracqui A, Kintz P, Ludes B. Buprenorphine-related deaths among drug addicts in France: a report on 20 fatalities. J Anal Toxicol 1998;22:430–4.
37. Amass L, Bickel WK, Higgins ST, Badger GJ. Alternate-day dosing during buprenorphine treatment of opioid dependence. Life Sci 1994;54:1215–28.
38. Amass L, Kamien JB, Mikulich SK. Efficacy of daily and alternate-day dosing regimens with the combination buprenorphine-naloxone tablet. Drug Alcohol Depend 2000;58:143–52.
39. Bickel WK, Amass L, Crean JP, Badger GJ. Buprenorphine dosing every 1, 2, or 3 days in opioid-dependent patients. Psychopharmacology (Berl) 1999;146:111–8.
40. Fudala PJ, Jaffe JH, Dax EM, Johnson RE. Use of buprenorphine in the treatment of opioid addiction. II. Physiologic and behavioral effects of daily and alternate-day administration and abrupt withdrawal. Clin Pharmacol Ther 1990;47:525–34.
41. Johnson RE, Eissenberg T, Stitzer ML, Strain EC, Liebson IA, Bigelow GE. Buprenorphine treatment of opioid dependence: clinical trial of daily versus alternate-day dosing. Drug Alcohol Depend 1995;40:27–35.
42. Cheskin LJ, Fudala PJ, Johnson RE. A controlled comparison of buprenorphine and clonidine for acute detoxification from opioids. Drug Alcohol Depend 1994; 36:115–21.
43. Nigam AK, Ray R, Tripathi BM. Buprenorphine in opiate withdrawal: a comparison with clonidine. J Subst Abuse Treat 1993;10:391–4.
44. Parran TV, Adelman CL, Jasinski DR. A buprenorphine stabilization and rapid-taper protocol for the detoxification of opioid-dependent patients. Am J Addict 1994; 3:306–13.

Chapter 4

Foreseeable Advantages and Limits of Buprenorphine-Naloxone Association

Michel Mallaret, Maurice Dematteis, Celine Villier, Claude Elisabeth Barjhoux, and Chantal Gatignol

1. INTRODUCTION

Drug addiction is a chronic, relapsing disease that results from the prolonged effects of drugs on the brain. Opioid dependence is a worldwide problem. In opioid-dependent humans, buprenorphine is an effective treatment alternative to methadone *(1,2)* and levomethadyl acetate hydrochloride *(3)*. The pharmacological profile of buprenorphine results in greater safety, less physical dependence, and greater flexibility in dose scheduling. However, abuse of buprenorphine has been reported in many countries where it is available as an analgesic *(4)* and in France *(5)*, where it is available as an opiate-analgesic for drug substitution and maintenance. Despite the partial agonist activity of buprenorphine at µ opioid receptors and its "ceiling effect", some cases of respiratory depression and fatalities have been reported, especially in cases of high doses of intravenously injected buprenorphine. The buprenorphine/naloxone (BupNx) combination tablet capitalizes on the differential absorption of naloxone by the sublingual (sl) vs parenteral routes: naloxone has a poor sl absorption. BupNx combination has been investigated with the goal of decreasing abuse, misuse, and diversion of buprenorphine. The BupNx combination product may be interesting for use in primary care office-based settings as a safe and an effective treatment that is likely to increase the availability

From *Forensic Science and Medicine: Buprenorphine Therapy of Opiate Addiction*
Edited by: P. Kintz and P. Marquet © Humana Press Inc., Totowa, NJ

of agonist treatment for opioid dependence. Availability of buprenorphine and BupNx tablets in United States has been slowed by the desire to provide them outside the traditional, highly regulated methadone clinic system. The Controlled Substances Act was amended in October 2000 and allows office-based prescribing of schedule III, IV, and V medications (and combination of medications) approved for opioid dependence and detoxification.

2. ADVANTAGES OF BUPRENORPHINE-NALOXONE ASSOCIATION

2.1. Advantages of Opiate-Naloxone Association: Lessons of the Past

2.1.1. Epidemic of Pentazocine and Tripelennamine Abuse in the United States

In the late 1970s an epidemic of abuse with "T's and Blues" began in which the opioid drug pentazocine-Talwin tablets (T) and the antihistamine tripelennamine (Blues) were crushed, dissolved together, and injected intravenously. The resulting "high" was reported to be similar to that of heroin. From 1977 to 1982, the iv use of the pentazocine/tripelennamine combination (Ts and Blues) had become a major drug abuse problem in St. Louis, MO. In 1983, the manufacturer of pentazocine tablets removed the drug from the pharmaceutical market and released a new tablet formulation of pentazocine and naloxone *(6)*. The Randall-Selitto and the hypertonic saline writhing tests studies, in two rat models, showed that a 100:1 dose ratio of pentazocine:naloxone was optimal and equivalent in oral analgesic effects to pentazocine alone. The same combination, administered parenterally to rats, showed little or no analgesia, indicating a suppression of pentazocine activity *(7)*. Consistently, 0.5 mg of naloxone hydrochloride, was added to the tablet formulation, this dose being inactive orally but active if administered parenterally (Talwin Nx). With these new tablets, there were only a few reports of abuse *(8,9)*. These residual cases of abuse may be owing to not only the psychostimulant effect of associated tripelennamine, but also to the lack of naloxone antagonism at opioid receptors (pentazocine is also an agonist at opioid receptors) and possibly to an unsufficient naloxone dose in Talwin Nx. However, since 1983, there has been a continuous decline in Ts and Blues abuse. The new pentazocine/naloxone tablets did not produce the euphoria sought by drug addicts. The Drug Abuse Warning Network in the United States and IMS America's National Prescription Audit reviewed the use and abuse patterns of pentazocine before and after the addition of naloxone in the pentazocine tablets. The rates of both emergency room and medical examiner mentions per million prescriptions were substantially lower during the 2 yr following the introduction of pentazocine/ naloxone tablets (decrease of 70% by emergency rooms and 71% by medical examiners) *(6,10)*. This decrease indicates that the product reformulation successfully reduced the abuse of pentazocine and its consequences.

2.1.2. Epidemic of Analgesic Buprenorphine Abuse in New Zealand

In 1990, New Zealand, there were considerable cases of iv injection of 0.2-mg tablets of analgesic buprenorphine with self-reports of misuse in 81% of the patients over the 4 wk prior to presentation to the Wellington Alcohol and Drug Centre *(11)*. Two surveys of 12-mo duration were undertaken on opioid users presenting to this center, before and after the introduction of a BupNx (0.2/0.17 mg) combination tablet. In the repeat survey, the reported misuse decreased; the BupNx tablet was subjectively less attractive and its street price was less expensive than buprenorphine's. One-third of the patients who used BupNx intravenously reported instances of withdrawal symptoms *(11)*. The cases of withdrawal symptoms after iv injection of BupNx suggest that most of these patients were buprenorphine dependent when they injected naloxone (and buprenorphine). The reduction in iv injection of buprenorphine, after the introduction of BupNX in New Zealand, was not total: however, few iv trials of BupNx by drug addicts followed the introduction of BupNx.

2.2. Buprenorphine and Naloxone: A Complex and Controversial Pharmacology

Buprenorphine is a partial agonist at μ opioid receptors and a low-efficacy partial agonist or antagonist at κ opioid receptors. At the δ opioid receptor, buprenorphine shows no agonistic activity (see review in ref *12*). Buprenorphine acts as a partial agonist at μ opioid receptors, which explains its high-affinity *(13)*, low intrinsic activity, and its slow dissociation at μ opioid receptors. Doses of buprenorphine necessary to obtain a ceiling effect are very different if buprenorphine is sublingually absorbed, intravenously injected, or intrathecally administered. A bell-shaped dose-response curve for buprenorphine has been described for its respiratory depression effect as well as for its antagonist effects *(14)*.

Recently, Bloms-Funke et al. *(15)* detected strong activities of buprenorphine at the nociceptin/orphanin FQ receptor (e.g., the human ortholog ORL1) using a receptor assay. Nociceptin is the endogenous ligand of the (opioid receptor-like) ORL1 receptor showing both hyperalgesic and antinociceptive properties in vivo. Buprenorphine behaves as a partial ORL1 agonist, which may contribute to its actions in pain models. The action of buprenorphine at the ORL1 receptor at higher concentrations may counter the antinociception produced by buprenorphine on opioid receptors, resulting in less nociception at higher doses and thus the bell-shaped dose-response curves. It is important to emphasize that the effects of buprenorphine on ORL1 receptors (which were investigated on induced inward currents in *Xenopus* oocyte potassium channels) are insensitive to naloxone *(15)*. In some cases *(16)*, the different effects of buprenorphine at these multiple receptors may explain how acute administration of naloxone incompletely antagonizes the effects of buprenorphine. In experimental studies of animals, continuous naloxone infusion increases the density of opioid-binding sites (upregulation) and potentiates behavioral responses to morphine, but the analgesic activity of buprenorphine is not modified, proving that nonopioid receptors are involved in buprenorphine analgesia *(17)*.

2.3. Clinical Aspects

Whether combined or not with naloxone in an sl tablet, buprenorphine has been shown to be effective in retaining patients in treatment and in reducing opioid use and craving, even when the tablets were dosed less than daily *(18,19)*. The pharmacological effects of buprenorphine are not altered by the addition of naloxone when sublingually administered to patients in an appropriate combination ratio. If BupNx is taken intravenously by patients, the decreased opioid effects and the withdrawal symptoms should reduce its abuse potential.

2.3.1. Pharmacokinetic/Pharmacodynamic Advantages of Associated Naloxone in BupNx Combination

Naloxone has a poor sl bioavailability, approx 10% *(20,21)*; the use of BupNx tablets by the therapeutic sl route produces a predominant buprenorphine effect. Concurrent iv administration of naloxone quickly attenuates the opioid effects of buprenorphine in opioid-dependent users *(22)*. Drug addicts look for the short-onset subjective effects of iv buprenorphine; iv naloxone decreases these effects.

Intramuscular naloxone challenge *(23)* produces withdrawal responses in buprenorphine-dependent patients: the latency to peak is shorter for im naloxone (0.5–2.0 h postinjection) than for per os naltrexone (3.0–4.0 h postingestion), a long-acting opioid antagonist. Naloxone, a short-acting opioid antagonist, has pharmacokinetic properties that allow a rapid decrease in subjective opioid effects and the short-term precipitation of withdrawal symptoms. These properties decrease the risk of illicit diversion and iv administration of BupNx tablets. The dose ratio of 4/1 (buprenorphine/naloxone: 8/2 and 2/0.5 mg) has been chosen: a dose ratio of 2/1 or 1/1 would induce too severe a withdrawal syndrome in the case of BupNx injection; a dose ratio of 8/1 would be unsufficient to avoid BupNx misuse and injection.

2.3.2. Sublingual Naloxone in BupNx Tablets Does Not Decrease Buprenorphine Effects

Strain et al. *(24)* compared buprenorphine (4, 8, and 16 mg) and BupNx tablets (1/0.25, 2/0.5, 4/1, 8/2, and 16/4 mg) in nondependent opioid abusers. Sublingual buprenorphine and BupNx produced the same profile of effects. These effects were similar to those of (im) hydromorphone (an opioid agonist; 2 and 4 mg), and, no significant differences were found between comparable doses of buprenorphine and BupNx. When 8-mg buprenorphine tablets were compared with 8/2-mg BupNx tablets, there was some attenuation of visual analog scale ratings of "liking", and "skin temperature", by naloxone, but these differences were small, nonsignificant, and not seen with other dose comparisons. In this study, sl naloxone did not attenuate sl effects of buprenorphine.

2.3.3. Sublingual Naloxone in BupNx Tablets Does Not Decrease Blockade Effects of Buprenorphine in Opioid-Dependent Patients

Buprenorphine, as a partial agonist at µ opioid receptors, usually blocks the effects of full agonists at µ opioid receptors. Buprenorphine thus reduces the number of heroin addiction relapses. Will naloxone decrease this therapeutic effect of buprenorphine? Hydromorphone challenges (12 mg intramuscularly) induced opioid agonist effects no matter what the escalating dose (4/1, 8/2, 16/4, 32/8 mg) of BupNx, but attenuation of the hydromorphone response occurred as the maintenance dose of BupNx increased. Maintenance on sl BupNx doses as high as 32/8 mg/d provides partial but not complete blockade to the acute effects of a complete opioid agonist (12 mg of hydromorphone intramuscularly) *(25)*. The minimal differences in blockade efficacy of BupNx at 1 vs 25 h after the maintenance dose show that naloxone does not modify blockade efficacy. This study demonstrates two important points: (1) the sl BupNx combination is not different from buprenorphine in blockade efficacy of abused or used opioid agonists, and (2) high sl naloxone doses do not alter opioid blockade by buprenorphine. In France, this buprenorphine property may delay but does not frequently limit the abuse of opiates by drug addicts. Sublingual BupNx tablets will probably not discourage such a use.

2.3.4. Sublingual Naloxone in BupNx Tablets Does Not Precipitate Withdrawal Symptoms in Opioid-Dependent Patients

Different doses of sl naloxone (0, 4, and 8 mg) in opiate-dependent volunteers stabilized on 8 mg of sl buprenorphine showed no evidence of precipitated opiate withdrawal *(21)*. Stoller et al. *(26)* showed that high doses of sl BupNx tablets (1/0.25, 2/0.5, 4/1, 8/2, and 16/4 mg) did not produce antagonist effects in hydromorphone-dependent (40 mg/d) patients. These results confirm the past hypothesis, pharmacokinetic data, and experimental clinical study results that the sl naloxone does not modify the potential of abuse of sl buprenorphine.

2.3.5. Is the BupNx Combination Effective for Detoxification or Treatment of Depressive Symptoms in Opioid-Dependent Patients?

Buprenorphine is widely used for maintenance, but it also has a potential utility to treat patients with opiate withdrawal syndrome. Opiate stabilization by BupNx (4/1 mg) tablets vs fixed-dose methadone (30 mg) was followed by lofexidine-assisted methadone withdrawal vs gradual BupNx reduction (1-mg reduction twice a week) in two groups of patients. Withdrawal symptoms in both groups were mild *(27)*. When compared to lofexidine, an $\alpha 2$ adrenergic agonist, and not to buprenorphine alone, sl naloxone from BupNx tablets does not seem to increase the withdrawal syndrome rate during detoxification of opioid-dependent patients.

Depression is frequent in opioid-maintained patients (rate as high as 50%) and is often associated with a poorer treatment prognosis. Branstetter et al. *(28)* showed that BupNx- or methadone-maintained patients experienced the same significant reduction in depressive symptoms (there was no control group). There was no significant difference in depressive symptoms no matter what the drug and the dose. Entering maintenance treatment has a positive impact on depressive symptoms, but in this study BupNx was not more effective than methadone.

2.3.6. What Is the Abuse Liability of Intravenous BupNx Combination in Nonopioid-Dependent and Opioid-Dependent Patients?

Many opiates are abused and injected by drug addicts. While BupNx tablets are water-soluble and available, these sl formulations have the potential to be injected. BupNx association will be advantageous if it induces no or few subjective opiate effects when BupNx is parenterally injected. Intravenous injection of BupNx may also precipitate a withdrawal syndrome.

2.3.6.1. Nonopioid-Dependent Abusers

Sublingual buprenorphine and BupNx induce subjective opiate effects *(24)* in nonopioid-dependent patients who may try to inject these tablets. Pickworth et al. *(29)* studied the subjective and physiological effects of iv buprenorphine (0.3, 0.6, and 1.2 mg) in nonopioid-dependent volunteers. Buprenorphine increased the scores on the Morphine-Benzedrine Group subscale of the Addiction Research Center Inventory. This effect was comparable with that observed *(30)* for iv morphine (20 mg/70 kg) or heroin (10 mg/70 kg). Buprenorphine induced euphoria and the visual analogous "good effects": these responses were similar to those of iv morphine (30 mg). The onset and increase in good effects, which are evident 5 min after injection, explain the potential of abuse of iv buprenorphine. While dissolving and injecting BupNx tablets should be aversive for opioid-dependent patients, the effects produced by Bup/Nx in opioid abusers who are not physically dependent are less clear. Weinhold et al. *(22)* showed attenuation of the effects of low-dose parenteral buprenorphine effects by parenteral naloxone.

2.3.6.2. Opioid-Dependent Abusers

If BupNx tablets were dissolved and injected by an opioid-dependent patient, then naloxone included in the combination should produce a precipitated withdrawal syndrome *(31–34)*. In opioid-dependent volunteers *(26)* who were maintained on 40 mg of oral hydromorphone, im BupNx (1/0.25, 2/0.5, 4/1, 8/2, and 16/4 mg) precipitated withdrawal symptoms; this effect was owing to naloxone and not to the partial agonist properties of buprenorphine at μ opioid receptors, since buprenorphine (8 mg) did not precipitate withdrawal symptoms in these patients. As withdrawal effects dissipated, euphoric opioid agonist effects from buprenorphine did not appear but pupil constriction occurred *(26)*. In another study *(19)*, iv BupNx was administered to opioid-dependent patients maintained with sl 8/2-mg BupNx tablets. During seven sets of four daily laboratory sessions, placebo, BupNx (4/1 and 8/2 mg), buprenorphine (4 and 8 mg), or hydromorphone (9 and 18 mg) was administered intravenously in a double-blind mixed order. During forced exposures, BupNx, buprenorphine, and hydromorphone produced dose-related increases in observer- and subject-rated agonist effects. After forced exposure sessions, the reinforcing effects of the drugs given on the past days were assessed in a multiplechoice session: subjects did not consistently identify these tested drugs as opiates, but all subjects chose hydromorphone and 8/2 mg of BupNx over saline in the drug-drug choices. The majority of subjects chose money over all drugs.

Naloxone included in BupNx tablets may have some advantages in opioid-dependent patients if iv naloxone precipitates withdrawal symptoms in these patients; these symptoms may decrease the BupNx abuse potential by the iv route. Naloxone challenges in humans maintained on a dose of buprenorphine used for treatment of opiate dependence demonstrated that buprenorphine induces physical dependence: naloxone precipitates reliable withdrawal in a dose-related way, as measured by subject-rated, observer-rated, and physiological measures. Nigam et al. *(35)* showed precipitated withdrawal when iv buprenorphine abusers (average of 1.33 mg/d) were challenged with 1.2 mg of naloxone intravenously. The magnitude of withdrawal syndrome produced by higher antagonist dose is substantial. In a residential laboratory study *(23)*, opioid-dependent volunteers were maintained on 8 mg/day of sl alcoholic solution of buprenorphine. They were challenged on independent occasions with placebo or im naloxone (0.3, 1, 3, and 10 mg/70 kg) after their daily buprenorphine dose using a repeated measures, crossover design. In this study, the naloxone dose needed to precipitate withdrawal was 10 higher than doses typically needed in morphine- or methadone-maintained patients. This need for a higher antagonist dose may be consistent with the presence of a relatively low level of physical dependence in buprenorphine-maintained humans. In a study by Eissenberg et al. *(23)*, the daily dose of buprenorphine was higher (8 mg/d sublingually) than the daily dose in a study by Kosten et al. *(36)*; (2 to 3 mg/day sublingually); for in these last data, the precipitated withdrawal occurred with a high dose of naloxone (35 mg/70 kg intravenously). The need for a higher antagonist dose may also reflect buprenorphine's complex pharmacology including its higher receptor affinity. The main goal of the BupNx association is not to induce severe withdrawal symptoms in drug addicts who inject BupNx. If this was the sole reason, a higher naloxone dosage in BupNx tablet would be necessary. The main goal of the BupNx association is in fact, to decrease the potential for buprenorphine abuse.

2.3.7. *Intravenous Naloxone May Decrease Respiratory Depression by Buprenorphine*

Buprenorphine is a partial opioid agonist with a ceiling effect with respect to respiratory depression *(37)*, when buprenorphine is sublingually absorbed. Lower doses of iv buprenorphine induce respiratory depression. In low opioid-dependent patients *(26)*, 10 mg of hydromorphone and 8 mg of buprenorphine intramuscularly induced a respiratory depression. Higher doses of associated buprenorphine and naloxone in 8/2 and 16/4 mg of BupNx intramuscularly and 8 mg of buprenorphine sublingually did not induce respiratory depression; naloxone antagonizes the respiratory depression induced by high doses of buprenorphine. In the case of iv administration of BupNx by drug addicts, naloxone would induce less respiratory depression than iv injection of a same dose of buprenorphine.

2.3.8. What Will Be the Epidemiological Consequences and Potential Economic Impact of the Use of BupNx Combination?

Epidemiological consequences of the use of BupNx combination by outpatients will be different in France, where buprenorphine is widely prescribed by general practitioners, and in the United States where only methadone is available and as a clinic-based treatment. In the latter case, if BupNx is widely available and correctly used, the number of somatic, psychological, and social complications induced by opiate abuse should decrease. Moreover, improving the accessibility, convenience, and acceptability of opiate substitution and maintenance therapy compared to clinic-based methadone maintenance will result in favorable economic consequences. The availability of take-home doses, without a high risk of diversion by injection, will decrease the cost of opiate maintenance. What is the economic impact of BupNx combination approval on office practice? In France, when available, the BupNx combination may decrease the buprenorphine black market, and an increasing number of patients who cannot be treated in methadone clinics may begin this therapy. For the United States, Rosenheck and Kosten *(38)* estimated the direct treatment cost compared with the clinic-based methadone cost, the relative effectiveness in reducing heroin addiction, health service use, crime and unemployment, and the ability to increase the number of maintained drug addicts. They estimated that costs of office-based treatment and clinic-based methadone treatment may be equivalent in the first year of treatment. The second year of treatment may generate annual savings of $400–600 per/patient. To the extent that BupNx combination is provided to previously unsuccessfully treated high-cost patients who usually receive several inpatient detoxifications each year, net cost savings could exceed several thousand U.S. dollars/annually per patient.

3. LIMITS OF BUPRENORPHINE-NALOXONE ASSOCIATION

3.1. Potential Risk of Inefficacy of Naloxone in BupNx Combination

Drug addicts often try to crush and heat tablets. They may also try to decrease naloxone's effects in different ways. (In France, in the 1980s, drug addicts could easily separate phenobarbitone from amphetamine associated in the same tablet for epileptic patients). In the BupNx combination, naloxone needs to be stable, no matter what adulterations drug addicts may use; no data have been published about naloxone's stability when these tablets are crushed, heated in a humid atmosphere, or exposed to ultraviolet rays. If stability decreases in one or several of these circumstances, the information will quickly spread among drug addicts and, consequently, iv injection and street value of adulterated BupNx tablets will increase dramatically. Nevertheless, the lack of large misuse or abuse of combinations of pentazocine and naloxone in the United States in the past and of analgesic doses of buprenorphine and naloxone in New Zealand may be partly reassuring, but some new misuses may always occur.

3.2. Abuse Liability of Intravenous BupNx Combination: Low But Still Possible

Will BupNx-maintained patients crush BupNx tablets and practice iv injection for subjective opiate effects? In some opioid-dependent patients *(19)* who were maintained with sl 8/2-mg BupNx tablets, intravenously injected BupNx (4/1 and 8/2 mg) did have low agonist opioid effects and did not precipitate a withdrawal syndrome; in these patients, opiate dependence may be lower than in patients maintained with hydromorphone *(26)*. The lack of precipitated withdrawal syndrome may be a reason to continue BupNx injection, even if the subjective effects of iv BupNx may be low. However, in a study by Stoller et al. *(26)*, after im BupNx injection, there was no subjective opiate effects (even if opiate pupil effects occurred). The hydromorphone-maintained patients did not present late subjective effects of buprenorphine (after the immediate withdrawal syndrome); the existence of pupil constriction proves that another agonist opioid effect occurred. It is not excluded that, in some patients, late-onset subjective effects of buprenorphine may induce an abuse, even if short-onset withdrawal signs and symptoms are aversive.

3.3. Adverse Buprenorphine Reactions and Sublingual BupNx Combination

Adverse buprenorphine reactions may occur when BupNx tablets are sublingually absorbed. In the French cases of buprenorphine fatalities *(5)*, buprenorphine was not always injected intravenously as suggested by some cases of great amounts of buprenorphine in the gastric contents and the absence of venipuncture. The physiopathological mechanisms of such fatalities are poorly understood. When (sublingually or intravenously) buprenorphine is abused, the cause of death may be respiratory depression, severe sleep disturbances (with associated central apnea), or possibly other toxic effects. With sl BupNx, naloxone is not absorbed and does not antagonize buprenorphine, so such fatalities might occur (even if they are rare).

3.3.1. Respiratory Depression

Intravenous buprenorphine injection is not the sole cause of respiratory depression. Ceiling effect is not constant. Respiratory depression, overdoses, and deaths from buprenorphine *(5)* have been reported, mainly in France, where more than 72,000 patients are maintained with buprenorphine treatment. These outpatients are mainly prescribed buprenorphine by generel practitioners. In patients who were hospitalized for buprenorphine respiratory depression or were found dead, iv buprenorphine injection was often diagnosed and associated benzodiazepines (or other psychotropic drugs) were frequently found. Respiratory depression was found for low doses of iv buprenorphine (1.2 mg) *(29)*, whereas higher sl buprenorphine doses are necessary to induce equivalent respiratory depression *(39)*. Intravenous buprenorphine injection has a higher potential for respiratory depression than sl buprenorphine. In many studies, naloxone decreases the respiratory depressant effects of postoperative buprenorphine, as it antagonizes pentazocine *(40)*. However, since buprenorphine has a high affinity for the µ opioid receptor, high doses of naloxone (5–10 mg) may be necessary to reliably reverse acute buprenorphine (0.3 mg/70 kg intravenously)-induced respiratory depression in humans or even may fail to reverse it. Buprenorphine also has a long elimination half-life and naloxone a short elimination half-life, so a single administration of naloxone may be unsufficient to antagonize secondary respiratory depression.

Respiratory effects of huge amounts of sl or intrathecal buprenorphine in humans are not well known. Even if there is a ceiling respiratory effect of an sl alcoholic solution of buprenorphine with doses ranging from 4 to 32 mg in nontolerant and nondependent volunteers *(39)*, this ceiling effect may not occur when buprenorphine is intrathecally or epidurally administered. In an experimental study *(41)*, buprenorphine abolished the fiber-mediated somatosympathetic reflex (lack of ceiling effect for C responses). Epidural administration of buprenorphine induced prolonged and biphasic respiratory depression *(42)*, sometimes resistant to naloxone *(16)*. If buprenorphine respiratory depression may be delayed during anesthesia *(43)*, this complication may occur during long-term treatment. It is important to emphasize that, in French fatalities *(5)*, brain concentrations of buprenorphine (a lipophilic drug) were up to 10-fold that of blood concentrations.

Ohtani et al. *(44)* and Huang et al. *(12)* have highlighted the role of the active metabolite of buprenorphine, norbuprenorphine, the *N*-dealkylated product of buprenorphine. Kuhlman et al. *(45)* as well as the monitoring of certain buprenorphine-maintained patients in France, demonstrated that the mean steady-state plasma concentration of norbuprenorphine exceeded that of buprenorphine after daily administration of sl buprenorphine to humans. Even if the intrinsic analgesic activity of intracerebroventricular norbuprenorphine is about one-fourth that of buprenorphine in the rat tail-flick test, norbuprenorphine does not cross the rat blood-brain barrier. Intravenous administration of norbuprenorphine at 1–3 mg/kg decreased respiratory rate, whereas buprenorphine had no effect up to 3 mg/kg. Norbuprenorphine induces respiratory depression, seemingly mediated by μ opioid receptors in the lung rather than in the brain *(46)*. In impaired renal function and renal failure, it is important to emphasize that blood levels of norbuprenorphine are increased by up to four times. Some associations with enzymatic inducer drugs induce hepatic microsomal enzymes called cytochrome P450 3A4 (oxidase). This effect may also increase formation of norbuprenorphine. In these cases or during a long-term treatment, norbuprenorphine may have a role in respiratory depression.

The frequent association with psychotropic drugs (e.g., alcohol, benzodiazepines, hypnotics, anxiolytics, antidepressants) in drug addicts may increase the effects of buprenorphine on respiratory depression. In most of the French fatalities, psychotropic drugs and mainly benzodiazepines were associated; benzodiazepines are known to dramatically increase experimental animal or human *(47)* buprenorphine respiratory depression.

3.3.2. Involuntary Overdoses

Because in France buprenorphine is widely prescribed for drug substitution or maintenance to outpatients, studies of adverse drug reactions show some cases of overdoses in children of patients who are maintained with buprenorphine. The BupNx tablets will induce the same risks for children of outpatients—naloxone, which is not sublingually absorbed, will not antagonize buprenorphine effects.

3.3.3. Experimental Buprenorphine Hepatotoxicity

In France, large overdoses or iv misuse of buprenorphine have caused hepatitis (unpublished data). Berson et al. *(48)* showed that buprenorphine (25–200 μM), and not norbuprenorphine, impaired mitochondrial respiration and adenosine triphosphate (ATP) formation in isolated rat liver mitochondria and microsomes, resulting in necrotic cell death. Four hours after administration of buprenorphine to mice (100 nmol/g of body wt), ATP was decreased and serum transaminase increased. Obviously, BupNx by either the sl or iv routes will not modify buprenorphine hepatotoxicity.

3.4. Specific Risks in Office-Based Treatment (BupNx Combination) of Opiate Dependence

Results of outpatient studies are often different from those of inpatient studies. Rapid tapering from heroin under various doses of sl buprenorphine or BupNx may produce moderate withdrawal symptoms occurring after initiation of buprenorphine treatment. The withdrawal symptoms may be owing to the antagonist effects of buprenorphine, an insufficient dose of buprenorphine, or confounding factors associated with continued street drug use. For these outpatients, there is a high risk of relapse of heroin use. The use of heroin during buprenorphine induction has an impact on the period required for stabilization. The sl BupNx combination includes the same risks that occur during buprenorphine treatment.

4. Conclusion

Buprenorphine is a high-affinity, partial μ opioid agonist and is approved as a pharmacotherapy for opioid dependence. Buprenorphine's ceiling effect on opioid agonist activity decreases the danger of overdose, may limit its abuse liability, and confers low toxicity even at high doses, increasing the dose range over which it may be safely administered. Buprenorphine may also produce sufficient tolerance and even block the effects of other opioids. Buprenorphine's slow dissociation from μ opioid receptors results in a long duration of action and diminishes withdrawal symptoms. Nevertheless, drug addicts frequently use the substance intravenously: the water-soluble tablets containing buprenorphine are crushed, dissolved and then injected. Deaths and severe respiratory depressions have occurred in France *(5)*. During recent years, however, there has been a reduction in the number of iv buprenorphine users as well as in the use or abuse of associated psychoactive substances, when the patients are included in maintenance programs *(49)*. There are still many iv buprenorphine abusers in France; ocular, skin, and soft tissue infections; viral hepatitis; autoimmune deficiency syndrome; and other diseases transmitted through drug injecting are frequent. To decrease the buprenorphine abuse liability, the combination BupNx tablet has been proposed in a dose ratio of 4/1 (8/2 and 2/0.5 mg).

Studies are needed on naloxone's stability so that not matter what adulterations drug addicts can imagine its stability will be maintained. Naloxone, a pure opioid antagonist, has a poor sl absorption. A BupNx tablet crushed, dissolved, and abused by injection will produce a predominant naloxone effect, because naloxone has good parenteral bioavailability. In this case, naloxone will decrease the effects of buprenorphine and produce a predominant opioid antagonist effect, in opioid-dependent and nonopioid dependent patients. An opioid-dependent patient who would experience the decrease in usual opioid effects or the precipitation of a withdrawal syndrome from injecting BupNx will presumably not abuse again this tablet by this route. Some complications will still occur with sl BupNx tablets: the adverse effects of high doses of sl buprenorphine will not be avoided by the poorly absorbed sl naloxone. Some of these adverse effects, including respiratory depression, will not be antagonized by the short-acting naloxone. Obviously, naloxone, a pure opioid antagonist, is ineffective at blocking the benzodiazepine increase of respiratory depression. In the case of BupNx abuse, hepatotoxicity of buprenorphine and adverse effects of sl buprenorphine will also still occur.

Buprenorphine is an effective medication that is useful for the treatment of opioid dependence. By adding naloxone to buprenorphine in the BupNx tablet, BupNx combination will be safer without inducing a too severe withdrawal syndrome in the case of iv injection; it may become a first-line treatment option for outpatients. It will be possible to prescribe take-home doses of BupNx tablets and to decrease the frequency of the risk of diversion and abuse by injection.

REFERENCES

1. Bickel WK, Stitzer ML, Bigelow GE, Liebson IA, Jasinski DR, Johnson RE. A clinical trial of buprenorphine: comparison with methadone in the detoxification of heroin addicts. Clin Pharmacol Ther 1988;43:72–8.
2. Johnson RE, Jaffe JH, Fudala PJ. A controlled trial of buprenorphine treatment for opioid dependence. JAMA 1992;267:2750–5.
3. Chutuape MA, Johnson RE, Strain EC, Walsh SL, Stitzer ML, Block DA, Bigelow GE. Controlled clinical trial comparing maintenance treatment efficacy of buprenorphine (bup), levomethadyl acetate (LAAM) and methadone (m). In: Problems of drug dependence, Harris LS, ed., NIDA Research Monograph. Washington, DC: US Government Printing Office, 1999.
4. Strang J. Abuse of buprenorphine. Lancet 1985;ii:725.
5. Tracqui A, Tournoud C, Kopferschmitt J, Kintz P, Deveaux M, Ghysel MH, Marquet P, Pepin G, Jaeger A, Ludes B. Intoxications aiguës par traitement substitutif à base de buprénorphine haut dosage. Presse Med 1998;27:557–661.
6. Baum C, Hsu JP, Nelson RC. The impact of the addition of naloxone on the use and abuse of pentazocine. Public Health Rep 1987;102(4):426–9.
7. Legros J, Khalili-Varasteh H, Margetts G. Pharmacological study of pentazocine-naloxone combination: interest as a potentially non abusable oral form of pentazocine. Arch Int Pharmacodyn Ther 1984;271(1):11–21.
8. Reed DA, Schnoll SH. Abuse of pentazocine-naloxone combination. JAMA 1986;256(18):2562–4.

9. Lahmeyer HW, Craig RJ. Pentazocine-naloxone: an "abuse proof" drug can be abused. J Clin Pharmacol 1986;6(6):389–90.
10. Poklis A. Decline in abuse of pentazocine/tripelennamine (T's and Blues) associated with the addition of naloxone to pentazocine tablets. Drug Alcohol Depend 1984;14(2):135–40.
11. Robinson GM, Dukes PD, Robinson BJ, Cooke RR, Mahoney GN. The misuse of buprenorphine and a buprenorphine-naloxone combination in Wellington, New Zealand. Drug Alcohol Depend 1993;33(1):81–6.
12. Huang P, Kehner GB, Cowan A, Liu-Chen LY. Comparison of pharmacological activities of Buprenorphine and norbuprenorphine: norbuprenorphine is a potent opioid agonist. J Pharmacol Exp Ther 2001;297(2):688–95.
13. Rosenbaum JS, Holford NH, Sdee W. In vivo receptor binding of opioid drugs at the mu site. J Pharmacol Exp Ther 1985;233(3):735–40.
14. Lizasoain I, Leza JC, Lorenzo P. Buprenorphine: bell-shaped dose-response curve for its antagonist effects. Gen Pharmacol 1991;22(2):297–300.
15. Bloms-Funke P, Gillen C, Schuettler AJ, Wnendt S. Agonistic effects of the opioid buprenorphine on the nociceptin/OFQ receptor. Peptides 2000;21(7):1141–6.
16. Knape JTA. Early respiratory depression resistant to naloxone following epidural buprenorphine. Anesthesiology 1986;64:382–4.
17. Paronis CA, Holtzman SG. Increased analgesic potency of mu agonists after continuous naloxone infusion in rats. J Pharmacol Exp Ther 1991;259(2):582–9.
18. Johnson RE, McCagh JC. Buprenorphine and naloxone for heroin dependence. Curr Psychiatry Rep 2000;2(6):519–26.
19. Amass L, Kamien JB, Reiber C, Branstetter SA. Abuse liability of IV buprenorphine-Naloxone, buprenorphine and hydromorphone in Buprenorphine-Naloxone maintained volunteers. Drug Alcohol Depend 2000;60(Suppl. 1):S6–7.
20. Preston KL, Bigelow GE, Liebson IA. Effects of sublingually given naloxone in opioid-dependent human volunteers. Drug Alcohol Depend 1990;25:27–34.
21. Harris DS, Jones RT, Welm S, Upton RA, Lin E, Mendelson J. Buprenorphine and naloxone co-administration in opiate-dependent patients stabilized on sublingual buprenorphine. Drug Alcohol Depend 2000;61(1):85–94.
22. Weinhold LL, Preston KL, Farre M, Liebson IA, Bigelow GE. Buprenorphine alone and in combination with naloxone in non-dependent humans. Drug Alcohol Depend 1992;30:263–74.
23. Eissenberg T, Greenwald MK, Johnson RE, Leibson IA, Bigelow GE, Stitzer ML. Burpenorphines physical dependence potential: antagonist-precipitated withdrawal in humans. J Pharmacol Exp Ther 1996;276(2):449–59.
24. Strain EC, Stoller K, Walsh SL, Bigelow GE. Effects of buprenorphine versus buprenorphine/naloxone tablets in non-dependent opioid abusers. Psychopharmacology 2000;148:374–83.
25. Strain EC, Walsh SL, Bigelow GE. Blockade effects of buprenorphine/naloxone combination tablet in opioid-dependent volunteers. Drug Alcohol Depend 2000;60(Suppl. 1):S216.
26. Stoller KB, Bigelow GE, Walsh SL, Strain EC. Effects of buprenorphine/naloxone in opioid-dependent humans. Psychopharmacology 2001;154(3):230–42.

27. Myles J, Law F, Raybould T, Singh S, Cockerill E, Nutt D. A double-blind randomized controlled trial of buprenorphine/naloxone (Suboxone) versus methadone/lofexidine for the detoxification of opiate-dependent addicts. Drug Alcohol Depend 2000;60(Suppl. 1):S156.
28. Branstetter SA, Kamien JB, Amass L. Methadone for the treatment of depressive symptoms in opioid-dependent adults. Drug Alcohol Depend, 2000; 60(Suppl. 1):S23.
29. Pickworth WB, Johnson RE, Holicky BA, Cone EJ. Subjective and physiologic effects of intravenous buprenorphine in humans. Clin Pharmacol Ther 1993;53(5):570–6.
30. Jasinski DR, Preston KL. Comparison of intravenously administered methadone, morphine and heroin. Drug Alcohol Depend 1986;17:301–10.
31. Preston KL, Bigelow GE, Liebson IA. Buprenorphine and naloxone alone and in combination in opioid-dependent human volunteers. Psychopharmacology 1988;94:484–90.
32. Mendelson J, Jones RT, Fernandez I, Welm S, Melby AK, Baggott MJ. Buprenorphine and naloxone interactions in opiate-dependent volunteers. Clin Pharmacol Ther, 1996, 60 : 105-14.
33. Mendelson J, Jones RT, Welm S, Baggott M, Fernandez I, Melby AK, Nath RP. Buprenorphine and naloxone combinations: the effects of three dose ratios in morphine-stabilized opiate-dependent volunteers. Psychopharmacology 1999;141:37–46.
34. Fudala PJ, Yu E, Macfadden W, Boardman C, Chiang CN. Effects of buprenorphine and naloxone in morphine-stabilized opioid addicts. Drug Alcohol Depend 1998;50:1–8.
35. Nigam AK, Srivastava RP, Saxena S, Chavan BS, Sundaram KR. Naloxone-induced withdrawal in patients with buprenorphine dependence. Addiction 1994;89:317–20.
36. Kosten TR, Krystal JH, Charney DS, Price LH, Morgan CH, Kleber HD. Opioid antagonist challenges in buprenorphine maintained patients. Drug Alcohol Depend 1990;25(1):73–8.
37. Walsh SL, Preston KL, Stitzer ML, Cone EJ, Bigelow GE. Clinical pharmacology of buprenorphine: ceiling effects at high doses. Clin Pharmacol Ther 1994;55:569–80.
38. Rosenheck R, Kosten TR. Buprenorphine/naloxone for opiate addiction: potential economic impact. Drug Alcohol Depend 2000;60(Suppl. 1):S187.
39. Walsh SL, Preston KL, Bigelow GE, Stitzer ML. Acute administration of buprenorphine in humans: partial agonist and blockade effects. J Pharmacol Exp Ther 1995;274:361–72.
40. Drummond GB, Fisher J, Zidulka A, Milic-Emili J. Pattern of reduction of ventilatory and occlusion pressure response to carbon dioxide by pentazocine in man. Br J Anaesth 1982;54(1):87–96.
41. Wang C, Chakrabarti MK, Whitwam JG. Lack of a ceiling effect for intrathecal buprenorphine on C fibre mediated somatosympathetic reflexes. Br J Anaesth 1993;71(4):528–33.
42. Molke Jensen F, Jensen NH, Holk IK, Ravnbord M. Prolonged and biphasic respiratory depression following epidural buprenorphine. Anaesthesia 1987;42(5):470–5.

43. McQuay HJ, Bullingham RES, Bennett MRD, Moore RA. Delayed respiratory depression: a case report and a new hypothesis. Acta Anaesthesiol Belgica, 1979;30(Suppl.):245–7.
44. Ohtani M, Kotaki H, Sawada Y, Iga T. Comparative analysis of buprenorphine-and norbuprenorphine- induced analgesic effects based on pharmacokinetic-pharmacodynamic modeling. J Pharmacol Exp Ther 1995;272:505–10.
45. Kuhlman JJ Jr, Lalani S, Magluilo J Jr, Levine G, Darwin WD, Johnson RE, Cone EJ. Human pharmacokinetics of intravenous, sublingual, and buccal buprenorphine. J Analyt Toxicol 1996;20:369–78.
46. Ohtani M, Kotaki H, Nishitateno K, Sawada Y, Iga T. Kinetics of respiratory depression in rats induced by buprenorphine-and its metabolite, norbuprenorphine. J Pharmacol Exp Ther 1997;281:428–33.
47. Kay B. Buprenorphine, benzodiazepines and respiratory depression. Anaesthesia 1984;39(5):491–2.
48. Berson A, Fau D, Fornacciari R, Degove-Goddard P, Sutton A, Descatoire V, Haouzi D, Letteron P, Moreau A, Feldmann G, Pessayre D. Mechanisms for experimental buprenorphine hepatotoxicity: major role of mitochondrial dysfunction versus metabolic activation. J Hepatol 2001;34(2):261–9.
49. Thirion X, Micallef J, Barrau K, Djezzar S, Lambert H, Sanmarco JL, Lagier G. Recent evolution in opiate dependence in France during generalisation of maintenance treatments. Drug Alcohol Depend 2001;61:281–5.

Chapter 5

Buprenorphine Maintenance Treatment in Primary Care

An Overview of the French Experience and Insight Into the Prison Setting

Marc Deveaux and Jean Vignau

1. INTRODUCTION

Buprenorphine has been proposed as a valuable substitution agent and a possible alternative to methadone for the treatment of opiate addicts because it has been shown to have a safer profile (less respiratory depression and sedation) and weaker withdrawal symptoms following abrupt discontinuation. Subsequently to the seminal report by Jasinski et al. *(1)*, many studies have been conducted to assess the possible use of buprenorphine to treat opiate-dependent subjects. Buprenorphine given sublingually to opiate-addicted subjects actually showed satisfactory clinical efficacy when compared to placebo *(2)*, impure placebo (i.e., low-dosage buprenorphine) *(3)*, and methadone *(4–6)*. However, the demonstration of buprenorphine's efficacy and safety also questions the legitimacy of the stringent regulations usually restricting opiate substitution treatments to a limited number of authorized centers. For 5 yr, French authorities have been the first in the world to decide to relax buprenorphine's legal control and to allow any physician and any community pharmacist to prescribe/deliver it to opiate-addicted patients.

From *Forensic Science and Medicine: Buprenorphine Therapy of Opiate Addiction*
Edited by: P. Kintz and P. Marquet © Humana Press Inc., Totowa, NJ

Many questions must be answered in order to help the possible extension of buprenorphine maintenance treatment (BMT) in primary care: Is buprenorphine provided in primary care relevant to the needs and expectations of drug users and their families? Is it safe? Is it accessible and acceptable? Is it effective in controlling opiate addiction and preventing subsequent relapses?

2. Implementation of BMT Through French Primary Care System

2.1. A Late But Considerable Concession to Harm Reduction Paradigm

While most European countries had promoted the use of methadone to treat opiate addiction, France remained firmly reluctant to give in to that mighty wave until 1995. Methadone programs then started to be implemented, slowly increasing the number of patients in treatment (up to 8000 in 2000) through registered addiction centers. One year later, in February 1996, BMT was made available at a large scale through the primary care system. The latter measure provoked distrust and indignation among those—social workers in their great majority—who had been traditionally involved in the rehabilitation of drug addicts through center-based drug free-oriented programs. General practitioners and pharmacists were speedily propelled on the front line of the treatment of opiate-addicted subjects. In 2000, they prescribed and delivered Subutex® (buprenorphine sublingual (sl) tablets, developed for maintenance treatment) to an estimated 80,000 patients. Parallel to the promotion of opiate substitution treatments, French authorities have allowed the sale of syringes by pharmacies since 1987 and have developed numerous (a hundred) needle exchange programs throughout the country since 1995.

2.2. Legal Framework of Therapeutic Use of Buprenorphine (7)

2.2.1. Essential Landmarks of French Health Services

France has a national health care service called Assurance Maladie, or Health Insurance (HI). That semipublic body was created just after the World War II and is paid for by national insurance. Almost every person is registered with one of the HI local agencies. As far as ambulatory medical care is concerned, most of the care providers (especially general and specialist doctors and pharmacists) are private professionals. Both practitioner's fee and medicament cost are charged to the patient. Subsequently, the latter is reimbursed by HI for about 70% of total expenses (in many cases the reimbursement is anticipated and the pharmacist only charges the remaining 30%). Many people also buy insurance to help pay for the remaining 30%. For those on low income, medical care is free.

2.2.2. Opioid Maintenance Treatments

Regulations ruling the prescription and delivery of Subutex are less restrictive than those applicable to methadone (narcotic schedule) but more stringent than those applicable to benzodiazepines (Table 1). Both buprenorphine and methadone are registered exclusively for long-term maintenance treatments and the patient must be over age 15. As for any narcotic drug, a prescription must be written after careful examination of the patient, on a special form designed to preclude forgery. This form is made of special watermarked paper and must bear the physician's name printed in blue and the patient's name, first name, age, sex, and address. The dosage must be written in words, not in figures (e.g., "Subutex eight mg/day, during twenty eight days") and must be dated and signed. It is also recommended that the prescribing practitioner and the patient support a therapeutic contract, in order to improve the patient's medical, psychological, and social condition.

Methadone maintenance treatment must be started by a physician belonging to a specialized center where various psychosocial services are available. Those centers are not governed by the HI system, which implies that their costs are actually borne by the state, and the patient has nothing to pay. After the patient is stabilized, the center can transfer methadone prescription and dispensation to a local general practitioner and pharmacist. Then, the habitual HI procedure is applied. Within either center- or office-based settings, methadone cannot be prescribed for longer than 14 d and take-homes are restricted to 7 d.

On the other hand, any physician, regardless of his or her discipline specialty, is allowed to initiate buprenorphine treatment, and any pharmacist is entitled to dispense Subutex. The prescriber is invited to write the name of the pharmacy where Subutex will be dispensed. Each prescription must not exceed 28 d. Prescription for shorter time periods are encouraged, and it is possible to demand daily delivery, under supervision of the pharmacist. Take-home doses are allowed for 7 d, or longer if expressly mentioned by the physician. The pharmacist must archive a copy of the prescription form for 3 yr. Daily dispensation on pharmacy premises is recommended during the first month of treatment.

Table 1
Comparison of Prescription and Delivery Regulations
of Buprenorphine, Methadone, and Benzodiazepines.

	Benzodiazepines	Buprenorphine	Methadone
Schedule	List I^a	List I^a	Narcotic list^e
Treatment induction by office-based physician	Allowed	Allowed	Not allowed
Prescription form	Ordinary paper	Special paper	Special paper
Maximal duration of prescription	28 d^b	28 d	14 d
Take-homes	28 d^{a,c}	7 d^d	7 d

^{a}Legal framework binding the delivery by the pharmacy of the listed medicines to a nominative prescription by a physician and excluding the possibility of renewable deliveries from initial prescription onward.
^{b}Except for flunitrazepam (14 d.)
^{c}Except for flunitrazepam (7 d).
^{d}Up to 28 d if expressly mentioned by the physician.
^{e}Legal framework adding the obligation for the physician to write his or her prescription on a paper designed to preclude from forging.

3. OBSERVABLE EFFECTS OF FRENCH POLICY

3.1. Is BMT Accessible and Acceptable?

The size of the population of patients under BMT is calculated from the number of Subutex boxes distributed monthly by wholesalers to the 23,000 French pharmacies, on the one hand, and the assumed average dosage per patient (fixed at 8 mg/d), on the other hand. The monitoring of Subutex sales has been entrusted to a national institute (Institut de Veille Sanitaire-InVS). This institute also monitors the sales of other health products (methadone, injection sets) meant for harm reduction in drug users and the occurrence of new human immunodeficiency virus-positive cases related to iv drug use. A recapitulative article was published in the InVS monthly bulletin concerning the 1996–1999 period *(8)*. Figure 1 shows the evolution of the estimated number of patients under BMT.

3.2. Is BMT Safe?

As a new substitution agent is made available for the treatment of drug addiction, the two main problems are its acute and chronic potential toxicity on the one hand and its possible diversion as a new addictive substance.

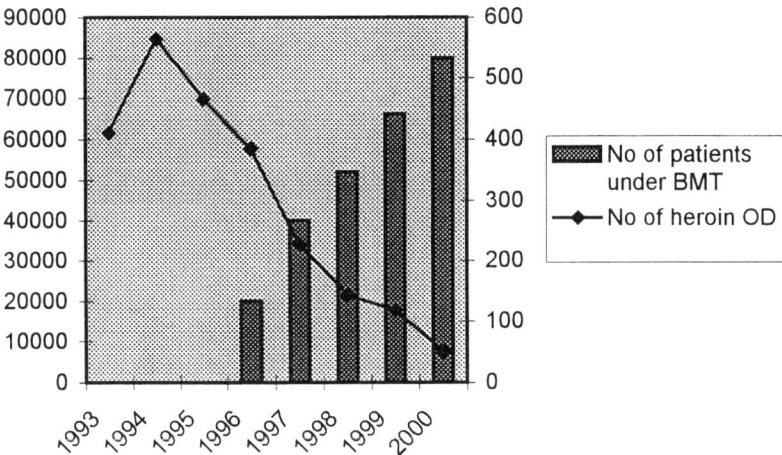

Fig. 1. Comparison between number of heroin overdoses (OD) and patients under BMT. (Adapted from ref. 8.)

3.2.1. Data from Preregistration Studies

3.2.1.1. Toxicity

As a partial agonist, buprenorphine exhibits a bell-shaped dose-effect curve, with intermediary doses producing stronger effects than higher ones *(9)*. That ceiling effect is observed for many of buprenorphine's physiological effects: anesthetic properties, responses of various autonomic functions such as respiratory depression, in particular *(10–13)*, and subjective effects *(14)*. Thanks to this ceiling effect, buprenorphine has been considered a potentially safe substitution agent.

3.2.1.2. Addictive Power

The reinforcing effects of buprenorphine were first evaluated in animals, using the self-administration method: "By definition, drugs that increase the probability of the behaviors that lead to their delivery are considered to act as reinforcers of behavior and to produce reinforcing effects" *(15)*. Drugs generating significant self-administration in animals are usually those that are abused by humans with a good correlation rate *(16,17)*. Assays designed to measure reinforcing effects of buprenorphine in several species showed a mild but real addictive power of that substance *(18,19)* subsequently confirmed in humans *(20)*. Note that buprenorphine was administered intravenously in all of these studies whereas buprenorphine available for opiate maintenance treatment is in sl tablet form. We now know the crucial role of pharmacokinetics in producing a reinforcing effect, i.e., the superiority of iv and pulmonary routes on the other ones *(21)*. Thus, we can reasonably speculate that addictive power of buprenorphine by the sl route is weaker than it is by the iv route.

3.2.2. Data from French Experience

3.2.2.1. Decrease in Overdoses

The growing use of buprenorphine has not paralleled an increase in overdose rate (Fig. 1). Conversely, overdose rate measured by the services of the French Ministry of the Interior (Office Central de Répression contre le Trafic et l'Importation de Stupéfiants) has shown an even and dramatic decrease since 1995 *(22,23)*. It is difficult to establish the exact role played by the widespread use of buprenorphine on this phenomenon. We suggest that a salient pharmacological feature of buprenorphine may explain its possible role in the decrease in overdoses. Actually, its kinetics of receptor occupation is characterized by an unusually slow dissociation *(24)* that makes it difficult for any concurrent agonist to displace buprenorphine from μ receptors. The presence of buprenorphine in the brain of an individual may thus protect him or her from opioid-agonist overdose.

3.2.2.2. Misuse

In the real world, outside the laboratory, the addictive power of a patent medicine can be indirectly estimated by the patterns of consumption it triggers in the population, especially the persistent and repeated attempts of addicted users to get more and more of the drug. In that respect, French HI has monitored the proportion of subjects who spontaneously consult more than one physician in order to cumulate a total amount far from the officially recommended dosage. (Almost the entire French population is affiliated with HI, a semipublic body. It is endowed with a new on-line procedure initially designed to faciliate the financial exchanges among patients, community pharmacies, and local HI agencies. This procedure also allows statistics.) A large body of evidence shows that the rate of simultaneous multiple consultation is remarkably low (ranging from 5 to 10%) when buprenorphine is considered *(25)*. By comparison, that rate is much higher for drugs with a well-known addictive power, such as flunitrazepam and high-dosage clorazepate. Differences in French regulation restrictions between buprenorphine and benzodiazepines are too small to explain this phenomenon. The reliability of the aforementioned HI data is particularly high since it is based on a substantial financial incentive in patients and pharmacists.

Sublingual Subutex tablets contain buprenorphine hypochloride salt and various excipients such as carbohydrate macromolecules (corn starch) and citric acid. Although such a formulation was designed to preclude iv deviation, some drug users found out a way to divert the tablets from therapeutic use. They crushed them, added water, let the mixture settle for a while, extracted the liquid upper layer by means of a syringe through a needle fitted with a filter, and eventually injected that suspension/solution. After 2 yr, such a deviation of buprenorphine tablets by drug users seems to range from 14 to 15%. These figures are based on direct interviews with drug users in different settings (e.g., ambulatory or residential addiction centers, inpatient addiction clinics, addictive medicine flying team within general hospitals) *(26)* and on interviews with physicians prescribing buprenorphine about their patients' injecting habits *(27)*. The reliability of these figures is fairly weak mainly because they are based on declarative data about a practice that is considered to be shameful and often hidden. A second bias is the questionable representativeness of the population samples assessed in the studies. The most readily accessible populations of drug addicts are those frequenting health care services. We know little about those addicts who are out of the scope of that system. Moreover, some components of the health system concentrate particular subpopulations whose unusual characteristics happen to be overrepresented in some studies.

3.3. Is BMT Effective in Controlling Opiate Addiction and Preventing Subsequent Relapses?

Three naturalistic studies of cohorts of French opiate-addicted patients under BMT have been published *(27–29)*. All three show a significant improvement in patients' medical, psychological, and social condition. None measured drug abstinence by urine toxicological testing. Vignau and Brunelle *(28)* prospectively compared BMT outcome in two groups of opiate-addicted patients treated within, respectively, office- or center-based settings ($n = 69$) for 24 wk. Using the Addiction Severity Index performed by a unique investigator, they observed a significant reduction in psychiatric comorbidity, family conflicts, legal problems, and alcohol and drug consumption in both groups. Compared with the two other studies, they found the poorest retention rate (72% at 6 mo for office-based-treated patients) and also the lowest buprenorphine dose per patient (mean dose ranging from 4.6 mg/d at entry into treatment to 5.9 mg/d after 6 mo). We suggest that these results are linked to each other, with chronic underdosage resulting in an increasing number of dropouts. De Ducla et al. *(29)* interviewed 71 general practitioners randomly recruited in four French cities about 300 patients under BMT. The physicians' opinion on BMT outcome was positive. They estimated that their patients had improved their occupational status, housing conditions, level of income, occurrence of deviant behaviors (such as prostitution, narcotic resale, and theft), and consumption of various psychoactive drugs. Duburcq et al. *(27)* prospectively interviewed 101 general practitioners about their patients ($n = 919$). They measured treatment outcome by monitoring prescribed daily dose of buprenorphine; rate of retention in treatment; TMSP addiction severity score (the TMSP score explores four dimensions of addiction severity: T-score is related to drug consumption; M-Score to medical problems; S-score to legal, social, and occupational problems; and P-score to psychiatric disorders caused by drug addiction); and Global Assessment of Functioning Scale (GAF-S) after 1, 3, 6, 12, 18, and 24 mo of BMT. Of the 919 patients included in the survey, 620 (67%) remained under the scope of health care services at the end of the observation period: five hundred eight (55%) continued to be treated by the initial physician, and 112 (12%) were treated by another physician or were referred to a hospital or an addiction center. Buprenorphine mean (SD) dose was 6.8 (5.7) mg/d at entry into treatment and 7.6 (5.4) mg/d at mo-24. However, from mo-1 assessment to mo-4 assessment, drug consumption decreased by 63%, and the use of iv route and TMSP scores also diminished (40%). Housing conditions, occupational activity, and GAF-S significantly improved.

4. PRISON

4.1. Drug Addicts in French Prisons

Officially, there are about 52,000 prisoners in France (96.2% male), and the mean incarceration time is 8.5 mo. Since 1994, each prison has been statutorily linked with a public hospital for health care provision *(30)*. Entering the prison, every detainee is registered with the local HI agency. This registration remains valid for 1 yr after release from prison. Although French prisons differ in the profile of the population incarcerated, the estimated proportion of drug-addicted subjects ranges from 17 to 50%. In Loos-lez-Lille prison, this proportion reaches about 50% of the 725 detainees *(7)*. Moreover, licit and illicit drug trafficking (mainly heroin and cannabis) cannot be avoided. Thus treating heroin abusers is essential in prison, in spite of a lack of consensus about the way to implement opiate substitution treatments. We describe next the work performed by the health care team of Loos-lez-Lille prison.

4.2. Legal Framework of BMT in Prison

Since December 1996, methadone and buprenorphine maintenance treatments could be started and continued in prison. In French prisons, methadone or Subutex, or both, are used. In some prisons, Subutex is readily and extensively offered to any detainee requesting that medication. In the great majority of the others, access to buprenorphine treatments is more strictly controlled (opiate addiction must be firmly established by clinical and toxicological tests). Subutex is prescribed monthly by a member of the prison's medical staff, then delivered by the prison's pharmacy and daily dispensed to the detainee under the supervision of a nurse.

In most of the French prisons, Subutex can also be obtained by between-inmate traffic or from visiting families. In 2001, the ongoing price of an 8-mg tablet sold on the black market is about equivalent 10–20 US dollars.

4.3. BMT Procedures in Loos-lez-Lille Prison

Concerning the procedures currently in use Loos-lez-Lille prison, we can isolate four different possibilities. The first procedure is applied to newcomers previously on BMT. At entry into jail, every newcomer is systematically examined by both a general practitioner and a psychiatrist. If the detainee declares he or she has been regularly treated by Subutex, BMT can be continued after confirming this by a phone call to his or her habitual physician or pharmacist. Psychosocial services are available along with the pharmacological treatment. The dosage may subsequently remain stable or gradually be decreased following a 10-d schedule *(31)*. The second procedure is applied to a newcomer not previously on BMT. Withdrawal syndrome may be treated using Subutex or nonopioid medicines. If used, Subutex is automatically discontinued according to a flexible dosing protocol. The third procedure is applied just before release from prison. Buprenorphine or methadone maintenance treatment can be started on detainee request during his or her stay in prison only at the end of it, in order to help prevent relapses after release from prison. Fourth is the case of drug addiction started during the stay in prison. Because of the importance of drug trafficking in jail, some detainees may become addicted to opiates during their stay. No procedure is relevant. In general, withdrawal symptoms are relieved by using pharmacological treatment, excluding the help of any opioid medication. Then, in the eventuality of repeated unsuccessful attempts by that method, BMT may finally be proposed.

A synopsis of the application of these different procedures in 1999 and 2000 is given in Table 2. The number of prisoners treated with buprenorphine has seen an almost exponential increase since 1996. The comparative variations in the numbers of patients treated with methadone and Subutex across the last 5 yr are shown in Fig. 2.

Table 2
Different Types of Buprenorphine Treatment
in Loos-lez-Lille Prison in 1999 and 2000[a]

	No. of patients	
Buprenorphine protocol	1999	2000
Fixed-schedule maintenance (8 mg/d)	102	206
Buprenorphine voluntary withdrawal	9	13
Treatment of opioid withdrawal syndrome[b]	90	80
Maintenance started before release from prison	20	10
Total	221	309

[a] Adapted from ref. 7.
[b] Gradual discontinuation of buprenorphine following a flexible 10-d schedule protocol.

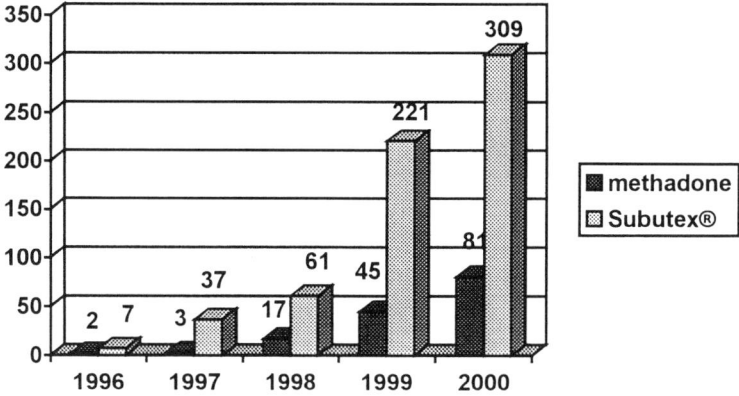

Fig. 2. Variations in the number of patients treated by either methadone or Subutex® across the last 5 yr in Loos-lez-Lille prison. (Adapted from ref. 7.)

5. CONCLUSION

The "French model" is worth thorough attention because it is the first attempt of a country to use high-dosage buprenorphine at a large scale, in the common, nonstigmatizing system of primary care (general practitioners and pharmacists). Legal guidance of therapeutic use is fairly liberal, which has made the treatment highly accessible. Because of the French welfare system, the cost directly borne by the patient is low or nonexistent. The major success of the implementation of this therapeutic policy is its positive impact on public health regarding its safety and feasibility. These encouraging results might not mask or underestimate the real difficulties encountered by primary care professionals and the development of buprenorphine misuse (especially the deviation to snorting and the iv route) and of its use in association with various psychotropic drugs (especially benzodiazepines) that may be hazardous. In prison, many impediments, mainly ideological, can be identified in order to implement evidence-based substitution treatment programs that match the real and important needs of the population incarcerated.

Acknowledgments

We wish to thank Catherine Adins and Ghada El Deeb for their help.

References

1. Jasinski DR, Pevnick JS, Griffith JD. Human pharmacology and abuse potential of the analgesic buprenorphine: a potential agent for treating narcotic addiction. Arch Gen Psychiatry 1978;35:501–16.
2. Johnson RE, Eissenberg T, Stitzer ML, Strain EC, Liebson IA, Bigelow GE. A placebo controlled clinical trial of buprenorphine as a treatment for opioid dependence. Drug Alcohol Depend 1995;40:17–25.
3. Ling W, Charuvastra C, Collins JF, et al. Buprenorphine maintenance treatment of opiate dependence: a multicenter, randomized clinical trial. Addiction 1998; 93:475–86.
4. Johnson RE, Jaffe JH, Fudala PJ. A controlled trial of buprenorphine treatment for opioid dependence. Jama 1992;267:2750–5.
5. Ling W, Wesson DR, Charuvastra C, Klett CJ. A controlled trial comparing buprenorphine and methadone maintenance in opioid dependence. Arch Gen Psychiatry 1996;53: 401–7.
6. Strain EC, Stitzer ML, Liebson IA, Bigelow GE. Comparison of buprenorphine and methadone in the treatment of opioid dependence. Am J Psychiatry 1994;151: 1025–30.
7. Deveaux, M, and Vignau, J. Prescription et dispensation de la buprénorphine haut dosage: bilan régional en médecine de ville et à la maison d'arrêt de Loos-lez-Lille [Prescription and delivery of high dosage buprenorphine: results in a region and in the Loos-lez-Lille jail]. Lett Pharmacologue 2001;15:4–8.
8. Emmanuelli J. Contribution à l'évaluation de la politique de réduction des risques SIAMOIS. Bulletin de l'Institut de Veille Sanitaire 2000;1:15–37.
9. Cowan A, Lewis JW, Macfarlane IR. Agonist and antagonist properties of buprenorphine, a new antinociceptive agent. Br J Pharmacol 1977;60:537–45.
10. Budd K. High dose buprenorphine for postoperative analgesia. Anaesthesia 1981;36:900–3.
11. Umbricht A. Safety of buprenorphine: no clinically relevant cardio-respiratory depression at high IV doses. In: Problems of drug dependence, 1998: proceedings from the 60th annual scientific meeting of the college on problems of drug dependence, NIDA Research Monograph Series (RM 179), National Institutes of Health, Rockville, MD, 1999.

12. Walsh SL, Preston KL, Bigelow GE, Stitzer ML. Acute administration of buprenorphine in humans: partial agonist and blockade effects. J Pharmacol Exp Ther 1995;274:361–72.
13. Walsh SL, Preston KL, Stitzer ML, Cone EJ, Bigelow GE. Clinical pharmacology of buprenorphine: ceiling effects at high doses. Clin Pharmacol Ther 1994; 55:569–80.
14. Huestis MA, Umbricht A, Preston KL, Cone EJ. Safety of buprenorphine: ceiling effect for subjective measures at high intravenous doses. In: Problems of drug dependence, 1998: proceedings from the 60th annual scientific meeting of the college on problems of drug dependence NIDA Research Monograph Series (RM 179), national Institutes of Health, Rockville, MD, 1999.
15. Negus SS, Woods JH. Reinforcing effects, discriminative stimulus effects, and physical dependence liability of buprenorphine. In: Buprenorphine: combatting drug abuse with a unique opioid. Cowan A, Lewis JW, eds., New York:Wiley-Liss, 1995, pp. 71–101.
16. Brady J V, Griffiths RR, Hienz RD, Ator NA, Lukas SE, Lamb RJ. Assessing drugs for abuse liability and dependence potential in laboratory primates. In: Methods of assessing the reinforcing properties of abused drugs, Bozarth MA, ed. New York: Springer-Verlag, 1987, pp. 48–86.
17. Yokel RA. Intravenous self-administration: response rates, the effects of pharmacological challenges, and drug preferences. In: Methods of assessing the reinforcing properties of abused drugs, Bozarth MA, ed., New York:Springer-Verlag, 1987, pp. 1–37.
18. Mello NK, Bree MP, Mendelson JH. Buprenorphine self-administration by rhesus monkey. Pharmacol Biochem Behav 1981;15:215–25.
19. Lukas SE, Brady JV, Griffiths RR. Comparison of opioid self-injection and disruption of schedule- controlled performance in the baboon. J Pharmacol Exp Ther 1986;238:924–31.
20. Pickworth WB, Johnson RE, Holicky BA, Cone EJ. Subjective and physiologic effects of intravenous buprenorphine in humans. Clin Pharmacol Ther 1993;53:570–6.
21. Mathias R. Rate and duration of drug activity play major roles in drug abuse, addiction, and treatment. NIDA Notes 1997;2:8–11.
22. Auriacombe M, Franques P, Tignol J. Deaths attributable to methadone vs buprenorphine in France. JAMA 2001;285:45.
23. Lepère B, Gourarier L, Sanchez M, Adda, C, Peyret E, Nordmann F, Ben Soussen P, Gieselbrecht M, Lowenstein W. Diminution du nombre des surdoses mortelles à l'héroïne en France depuis 1994: à propos du rôle des traitements de substitution. Ann Med Interne (Paris) 2001;152:5–12.
24. Boas RA, Villiger JW. Clinical actions of fentanyl and buprenorphine: the significance of receptor binding. Br J Anaesth 1985;57:192–6.
25. Cholley D, Weill G. Traitement de substitution par buprenorphine haut dosage. Concours Méd 1999;121:1552–4.
26. Thirion X, Barrau K, Micallef J, Haramburu F, Lowenstein W, Sanmarco JL. Traitement de substitution de la dépendance aux opiacés dans les centres de soins: le programme OPPIDUM des Centres d'Evaluation et d'Information sur la Pharmacodépendance. Ann Med Interne (Paris) 2000;151(Suppl. A):A10–7.

27. Duburcq A, Charpak Y, Blin P, Madec L. Suivi à 2 ans d'une cohorte de patients sous buprénorphine haut dosage. Résultats de l'étude SPESUB. Rev Epidemiol Santé Publique 2000;48:363–73.
28. Vignau J, Brunelle E. Differences between general practitioner- and addiction centre- prescribed buprenorphine substitution therapy in France. Preliminary results. Eur Addict Res 1998;4:24–8.
29. De Ducla M, Gagnon A, Mucchielli A, Robinet S, Vellay A. Suivi de patients pharmacodépendants aux opiacés traités par buprénorphine haut dosage à partir de réseaux de soins: étude rétrospective nationale. Ann Med Interne (Paris) 2000;151(Suppl. A):A27–32.
30. Hedouin V, Luneau E, Revuelta E, Becart A, Deveaux M, Gosset D. An aspect of clinical forensic medicine in France: health care to jail detainees. In: Proceedings of the 49th Annual Meeting of the American Academy of Forensic Sciences, Armstong, ed., Colorado Springs, CO:McCormick, 1997.
31. Vignau J. Preliminary assessment of a 10–day rapid detoxification programme using high dosage buprenorphine. Eur Addict Res 1998;4:29–31.

Chapter 6

Buprenorphine as a Viable Pharmacotherapy in Australia

John H. Lewis

1. INTRODUCTION

Australia, like many other countries, has witnessed a significant increase in opioid-dependent persons since the mid-1960s, when it first became apparent that there was a need for treatment facilities. Australia's first drug referral center opened in Sydney in 1964 as a drop-in counseling service. Following the pioneering work of Dole and Nyswander *(1)* in the use of methadone blockade in the United States, in 1969 Dalton et al. *(2)* introduced methadone into Australia as an opiate substitute. In the mid-1980s, methadone maintenance units opened up offering a range of counseling services in addition to daily methadone dosing. Methadone has continued to be the treatment of choice, with client numbers increasing from 2000 in 1985 to 26,000 in 2000. On a population basis, Australia has a higher number of clients per million inhabitants than either the United States or the United Kingdom.

Despite the uptake of methadone as a cost-effective maintenance therapy, there have been many problems with diversion and injection of take-home doses *(3,4)*. There have been deaths from methadone toxicity, either at commencement of dosing or through self-administration *(5,6)*. Zador et al. *(7)* reported on 211 deaths among persons enrolled in New South Wales (NSW) methadone programs between 1990 and 1995. In a study of 242 methadone-related deaths in NSW programs in that same period, Sunjic et al. *(8)* noted that 10% of opioid overdoses involved methadone syrup and the remainder a combination of syrup and tablets. They found that 72 of these deaths were from persons enrolled in methadone maintenance treatment at the time.

From *Forensic Science and Medicine: Buprenorphine Therapy of Opiate Addiction*
Edited by: P. Kintz and P. Marquet © Humana Press Inc., Totowa, NJ

Since its inception as an opiate substitute, methadone has been plagued by bad publicity, insufficient placement in programs, and inadequate supervision facilities in many existing clinical practices. The stigma associated with methadone treatment has been a major factor in deterring opioid-dependent people from seeking treatment. The lack of alternative treatments and high level of bureaucratic regulation have contributed to the negativity surrounding methadone. Compounding these problems, there have been a number of deaths during induction into methadone treatment, and overdose deaths as a result of methadone syrup being diverted and sold on the black market. Finally, a significant proportion of methadone-maintained subjects experience difficulties with side effects. Apart from these negative aspects of methadone, Australia has witnessed a rise in opioid-related deaths from 45 per million population in 1988 to 112 per million population in 1998 *(9)*. For all these reasons, there is a great need for alternative pharmacotherapies for opioid dependence, particularly alternatives with a wider margin of safety *(10)*.

2. BUPRENORPHINE

There have been Australian trials of the three major alternative pharmacotherapies: naltrexone, levomethadyl acetate, and buprenorphine. Buprenorphine has been the most extensively studied. The drug has been available in Australia since 1983 as Temgesic®. Originally an S4 schedule (prescription only) and approved only as an analgesic, buprenorphine was rescheduled in 1992 as an S8 (drug of addiction). In the mid-1980s, there was some abuse of Temgesic in Western Australia, prompting studies into its potential as an opiate substitute.

Seow et al. *(11)* conducted early clinical trials in Western Australian into the use of buprenorphine as a maintenance agent for opiate-dependent outpatients. They assessed the acceptability of 2–4 mg of daily sublingual (sl) buprenorphine in a group of heroin-dependent subjects and the effects of abrupt withdrawal and subsequent reintroduction. All subjects ($n = 32$) in this study were given either a 2- or 4-mg daily sl dose in an alcohol/buffered preparation in wk 1, 2, 4, and 5 with a placebo in wk 3. Urinalysis was conducted for abused drugs. The study demonstrated that although buprenorphine was well tolerated by the subjects, they all experienced the maximum number of withdrawal symptoms during the placebo week and there was no drop in opiate-positive urines throughout the period. The investigators concluded that an sl dose >4 mg was required if buprenorphine was to be used in maintenance therapy.

In a subsequent double-blind study, Quigley et al. *(12)* assessed the effect of gradual detoxification in outpatient addicts who had been stabilized on 4 mg of sl buprenorphine daily. Heroin addicts with a history of buprenorphine abuse were stabilized on 4 mg of sl buprenorphine daily for 14 d followed by a double-blind gradual detoxification and subsequent placebo for 2 wk thereafter. Using criteria similar to those of the previous study *(11)*, Quigley et al. *(12)* concluded that using a 4-mg dose of buprenorphine, subjects experienced unacceptable detoxification symptoms and poor abstinence from other opiates. The study reaffirmed the need for future trials of buprenorphine using a higher daily dose of 8 or 16 mg. Little other research into buprenorphine was conducted until the mid-1990s, when it became apparent that more comprehensive investigation was needed into the practicality of introducing buprenorphine into the community. Renewed interest in buprenorphine hinged on four key properties of the drug: its safety; poor oral bioavailability, posing a low risk of overdose; lower respiratory depression; and the option of second daily dosing.

Australia's record of providing adequate drug treatment and a commitment to minimization of harm, including needle exchange facilities, paved the way for one of the largest randomized controlled trials of buprenorphine ever conducted. The value of buprenorphine to Australia was in maintenance therapy and in withdrawal from both heroin and methadone. Mattick et al. *(13)* have well reviewed a comprehensive critique of earlier clinical trials involving buprenorphine. Previous randomized controlled trials have been limited by dose ranges, fixed doses, and the use of ethanol-based liquid rather than tablets *(14,15)*.

The National Drug and Alcohol Research Centre, University of New South Wales, coordinated a randomized trial of buprenorphine vs methadone maintenance from 1996 to 1997 *(16)*.

The multisite 13-week trial recruited 405 heroin-dependent patients at three sites (two in Sydney, one in Adelaide). The study was double blind and double dummy. It used flexible dosing 2–32 mg of sl buprenorphine or 20–150 mg methadone syrup. Alternate-day dosing of active buprenorphine under double-blind conditions was implemented. Patients provided urine samples to test for opiate and polysubstance abuse.

The study concluded, among other things, that buprenorphine and methadone were equivalent in patient retention and suppression of heroin use as well as in suppressing other drug use and reducing the risk of human immunodeficiency virus. Furthermore, alternate double-day dosing was effective in 85% of patients maintained on this regimen. The majority of patients were effectively maintained on 8 mg daily or 16 mg second daily dosing.

An important aspect of this study was the flexible dose setting, so that basically patients set their own doses. One consequence of this was that many patients settled for quite low doses, and the average maintenance dose of buprenorphine was <8 mg. It has previously been observed in methadone treatment that many patients settle for suboptimal doses and have to be encouraged to taker higher and more effective daily doses. In this study, it is possible that outcomes would have been better had some patients been encouraged to receive higher doses of buprenorphine.

3. National Evaluation of Pharmacotherapies for Opioid Dependence

In 1998, the Australian federal government launched a 3-yr national evaluation project the National Evaluation of Pharmacotherapies for Opioid Dependence (NEPOD), to investigate pharmacotherapies as treatment options for maintenance, withdrawal, and relapse prevention in opioid dependence *(16)*. In part, the NEPOD *(17)* project was in response to widespread community and political support for making naltrexone widely available. Several state governments funded trials of naltrexone treatment, and the NEPOD project was designed to ensure the optimal scientific evaluation by being able to compare the results of many trials. NEPOD facilitates collaboration among research groups conducting trials, monitors and analyzes core data sets, and coordinates an assessment of the relative cost-effectiveness of these pharmacotherapies. Most previously published studies have focused on the role of buprenorphine as a maintenance therapy. However, the drug has been identified as being useful in the management of opioid withdrawal, and, thus, a number of NEPOD projects are being conducted in order to evaluate this potential role. Some of the Australian trials involving buprenorphine are given in Table 1.

4. Conclusion

Currently, Australian governments are preparing for the implementation of buprenorphine treatment. The National Expert Advisory Committee on Illicit Drugs has the role of formulating guidelines on the use of buprenorphine. Strategies for dosing within clinics, distribution in retail pharmacies, patient monitoring, and the possibilities of diversion and overdose have been discussed at the state level, and policies are being implemented. Buprenorphine is expected to be of special value in prisons. In this context, where history can be difficult to verify, the greater safety of buprenorphine during induction into treatment makes it a preferable drug to methadone.

Table 1
Australian Trials on Buprenorphine

Trial	Status
Methadone withdrawal using buprenorphine	Completed
Buprenorphine-assisted withdrawal vs conventional detoxification	Completed
Inpatient buprenorphine dosing study	Completed
Inpatient buprenorphine withdrawal dosing study followed by naltrexone	Completed
Buprenorphine treatment for Vietnamese heroin users	Completed
Randomized control trial of buprenorphine-assisted detoxification from heroin in specialist and primary care settings	Current
Buprenorphine detoxification in specialist vs primary care settings	Current
Buprenorphine-assisted withdrawal vs methadone withdrawal	Current
Randomized control trial of buprenorphine vs clonidine in detoxificiation from heroin	Current
Buprenorphine-assisted detoxification in correctional centers	Proposed

The role of buprenorphine in Australia as an alternative to existing treatments, particularly methadone, will not be known for some time. There appears to be consensus on the need for higher rather than lower doses. However, implementation of high doses may ultimately depend on the patient's ability to pay unless the drug is placed under the Pharmaceutical Benefits Schedule. The relatively high cost (AUD$4–5) per tablet, long dosing time (4 min), and patient acceptance and compliance will become the most significant determinants as to the long-term future of the use of buprenorphine in Australia.

Acknowledgments

Appreciation is expressed to Dr. James Bell, director of Drug and Alcohol Services, South East Area Health Services, Sydney, and to Associate Professor Richard Mattick of the National Drug and Alcohol Research Centre, University of New South Wales for their valuable advice and access to research data.

References

1. Dole VP, Nyswander M. A Medical Treatment for diacetylmorphine (heroin) addiction. JAMA 1965;193(8):646–50.
2. Dalton MS, Duncan D, Taylor N. Methadone blockade in the treatment of opiate addiction: a follow-up study. Med J Aust 1976;20:755–6.
3. Darke S, Ross J, Hall W. Prevalence and correlates of the injection of methadone syrup in Sydney, Australia. Drug and Alcohol Dependence 1996;43:191–8.

4. Lintzeris N, Lenne M, Ritter A. Methadone injecting in Australia: a tale of two cities. Addiction 1999;94(8):1175-8.
5. Drummer OH, Syrjanen M, Opeskin K, Cordner S. Deaths of heroin addicts starting on a methadone maintenance programme. Lancet 1990;335:108.
6. Drummer OH, Opeskin K, Syrjanen M, Cordner SM. Methadone toxicity causing death in ten subjects starting on a methadone maintenance program. American Journal of Forensic Medicine and Pathology 1992;13:346-50.
7. Zador D, Sunjic S, Basili H. Deaths in methadone maintenance treatment in New South Wales, 1990-1995. In: Hall W, ed, Proceedings of an international opioid overdose symposium. National Drug and Alcohol Research Centre Monograph no. 35. Sydney: National Drug and Alcohol Research Centre, 1998.
8. Sunjic S, Zador D, Basili H. Methadone-related deaths in New South Wales. July 1990-December 1995. In: Hall W, ed, Proceedings of an international opioid overdose symposium. National Drug and Alcohol Research Centre Monograph no. 35. Sydney: National Drug and Alcohol Research Centre, 1998.
9. Australian Bureau of Statistics data on opioid overdoses. Canberra Australia, 1999, found at www.med.unsw.edu.au/ndarc/questions/overdosedata.htm.
10. Ali RL, Quigley AJ. Accidental drug toxicity associated with methadone maintenance treatment. Med J Aust 1999;170:100-1.
11. Seow S, Quigley A, Ilett K, Dusci L, Swensen G, Harrison-Stewart, Rappeport L. Buprenorphine: a new maintenance opiate? Med J Aust 1986;144:407-11.
12. Quigley A, Seow S, Ilett K, Dusci L, Swensen G, Harrison-Stewart, Rappeport L. Buprenorphine: detoxification after maintenance treatment. Aust Drug Alcohol Review 1987;6:5-10.
13. Mattick RP. In: Methadone maintenance treatment and other opioid replacement therapies, Mattick RP, Oliphant D, Ward J, Hall W, eds., Amsterdam: Harwood Academic, 1988.
14. Bickel WK, Stitzer ML, Bigelow GE, Liebson IA, Jasinski DR, Johnson RE. A clinical trial of buprenorphine: comparison with methadone in the detoxification of heroin addicts. Clin Pharmacol Ther 1988;43:72-8.
15. Johnson RE, Jaffe JH, Fudala PJ. A controlled trial of buprenorphine treatment for opioid dependence. JAMA 1992;267(20):2750-5.
16. Mattick RP, Ali R, White J. A comparative study of buprenorphine and methadone in the treatment of opioid dependence. Research Protocol. Sydney, Australia: National Drug and Alcohol Research Centre, University of New South Wales 1999.
17. National evaluation of pharmacotherapies for opioid dependence (NEPOD). National Drug and Alcohol Research Centre, University of New South Wales, Sydney, Australia, 1998.

Chapter 7

Separative Techniques for Determination of Buprenorphine

Vincent Cirimele

1. INTRODUCTION

Buprenorphine was initially developed for the treatment of acute and chronic pain, especially of surgical or neoplastic origin. However, the drug presents some addiction potential and cases of abuse have been reported in France. As a consequence, it has become necessary for clinical and forensic laboratories to be able to assay buprenorphine in biological samples. This determination is, however, difficult, owing to the very low therapeutic plasma concentrations.

Immunoassay offers rapid and sensitive identification of buprenorphine that is well adapted to general, unknown screening situations. However, the technique suffers from interferences and does not allow the separate quantitation of buprenorphine and norbuprenorphine. Since the first published report on buprenorphine determination in plama in 1980 *(1)*, a wide range of techniques have been proposed—including thin-layer chromatography (TLC); high-performance liquid chromatography with ultraviolet (HPLC-UV), fluorometric, electrochemical, and mass spectrometric detection; and gas chromatography (GC) with nitrogen-phosphore, electron-capture, and mass spectrometric detection—for the determination of buprenorphine in biological samples (blood, urine, bile, gastric content, tissus, feces), but also in alternative specimens such as hair or sweat.

The aim of this chapter is to review the existing separative techniques for the determination of buprenorphine in biological specimens and to discuss the performance of these methods in terms of both sensitivity and specificity.

From *Forensic Science and Medicine: Buprenorphine Therapy of Opiate Addiction*
Edited by: P. Kintz and P. Marquet © Humana Press Inc., Totowa, NJ

2. DETERMINATION OF BUPRENORPHINE IN BLOOD

The first report on buprenorphine determination in plasma was published in 1980 *(1)*. Buprenorphine was injected into baboons (5 mg/kg), and plasma was extracted using a complex liquid-liquid extraction (LLE) to limit the interfering peaks. Gas chromatography/mass spectrometry (GC/MS) was used, and the monosilyl derivative with BSA, obtained after heating at 40°C for 15 min, was analyzed. This method is delicate, time-consuming, and leads to low recovery owing to the multiple LLE steps. In the single-ion monitoring (SIM) mode of detection, a limit of detection (LOD) of 20 ng/mL was obtained.

In 1985, Tebbett *(2)* described HPLC-UV method for determining buprenorphine in serum after extraction with diethyl ether in alkaline conditions. After separation on a 5-µm Supelco RP-18 column (200 x 4.5 mm id), detection was achieved at 290 nm. The high extraction rate (98–100%) and the limited sensitivity (1 ng/mL) of the outlined method were found to be suitable for the determination of buprenorphine in the serum of patients receiving high doses of the drug or in blood samples obtained from buprenorphine abusers. Similar performances were observed by Lagrange et al. *(3)* using a two-step LLE (hexane-isopropyl alcohol in alkaline conditions and back-extraction in acid). Accurate quantification was obtained using clothiapine as internal standard after detection at 214 nm. For two patients who started a maintenance program by sublingual (sl) form, buprenorphine concentrations were 32 and 45 ng/mL in plasma. These patients were admitted in an emergency department for coma, and the administered dose and route were unknown. In a third case, the concentration of buprenorphine was 4 ng/mL.

The HPLC assay with fluorescence detection (excitation: 285 nm, emission: 350 nm) developed by Garrett et al. *(4)* was able to detect a concentration of 5 ng/mL using a two-step extraction procedure. A better sensitivity (1 ng/mL) was obtained by Ho et al. *(5)* after extraction of plasma with hexane-isoamyl alcohol at pH 9.25 and detection at 345 nm (excitation 210 nm). Owing to its greater selectivity, the reversed-phase chromatography on a µPorasil column (300 x 2 mm id) permitted the first pharmacokinetic study of iv buprenorphine (6 mg/kg) for pain relief in a 45-yr-old female patient after thyroid goiter resection. Plasma concentration-time profile decreased from 102 to 1.1 ng/mL in 220 min after injection.

In the previous HPLC methods, detection limits were in the nanograms/milliliter range (1–5 ng/mL). Lower LOD was reached (40 pg/mL) with the column-switching solid-phase trace-enrichment HPLC method followed by electrochemical detection (ECD). The procedure developed by Schleyer et al. *(6)* involves a solid-phase extraction (SPE) on an LC_{18} 40-µm SuperClean column; a LiChroCART 4 × 4 mm RP-18 cartridge containing 5 µm of C_{18} material to concentrate 50 repetitive injections of plasma; and a 30 × 4 mm id, 5-µm particle size C_{18} cartridge for the chromatography. The most sensitive detection was achieved when the electrode voltage was set at 480 mV. Thirty minutes after sc injection of buprenorphine into six patients, the concentration of buprenorphine in plasma was 2.9 ng/mL on average. For the patients receiving sl application, the average plasma concentration was 250 pg/mL. Norbuprenorphine was detectable in the plasma of these patients with an average concentration of 60 pg/mL. The concentration-time curves for buprenorphine obtained from two patients after sc application of 5 µg/kg body wt buprenorphine showed decreasing concentrations from 4865 and 2357 ng/mL (peak concentration) to 50 pg/mL for the two subjects, respectively. This procedure was proposed for broad clinical use and for the monitoring of drug levels during therapeutic interventions.

In 1990, Martinez et al. *(7)* published a comparative study for the identification and determination of buprenorphine in plasma, based on GC with two detectors. For purification, the diluted and alkalinized plasma (pH 9.2) was deposited on an Extrelut-20 column. The diethyl ether eluate was evaporated and the dry residue redissolved in acetic anhydride-pyridine (1:1) or in heptafluorobutyric anhydride. In both cases, chromatographic separation was obtained on the same column (OV-1 column, HP-1, 5 m × 0.530 mm id), but detection was achieved on nitrogen-phosphorus detector (NPD) for acetyl derivatives and ECD for heptafluorobutyryl derivatives. Limits of detection were 0.5 and 50 ng/mL for the heptafluorobutyryl and acetyl derivatives, respectively. The investigators concluded that the determination of the drug at therapeutic or subtherapeutic levels was advisable by GC/ECD, but no clinical application was presented. Only qualitative determination of buprenorphine in plasma of rats after iv administration of 0.6 mg was given as an example. In fact, this method, requiring 2–4 mL of plasma, does not achieve the desired limit of quantification.

By refining the extraction and derivatization procedure of Cone et al. *(8)*, Everhart et al. *(9)* developed a method for the measurement of buprenorphine in plasma with a limit of quantification of 100 pg/mL. Plasma (1 mL) was extracted using a four step procedure: ethyl acetate/heptane 4:1 [v/v] at pH 9.13; sulfuric acid; toluene:*t*-amyl alcohol (9:1 [v/v]); and, finally, ethyl acetate/heptane (4:1 [v/v]) at pH 9.13. The heptafluorobutyric derivative (toluene/heptafluorobutyric anhydride, 2:1 [v/v]; was analyzed by GC/ECD using an Ultra-1 fused-silica capillary column (25 m × 0.2 mm id). This method was used in human pharmacokinetics to study the bioavailability of different formulations. Buprenorphine concentrations were in the range of 0.2–14.3 ng/mL.

Some modifications were adopted in comparison with the previously published method by Cone et al. *(8)*. For example, the pH was maintained at the isoelectric point during the extraction procedure to maximize recovery, the tubes used for derivatization were silanized to minimized decomposition, more stable heptafluorobutyryl esters were obtained (instead of pentafluoropropyl esters), microvial inserts were deactivated to prevent adsorption of the derivatives of buprenorphine and modern capillary GC instead of packed-column chromatography was used.

In 1985, Blom et al. *(10)* published the first method with sufficient specificity and sensitivity for the characterization of the clinical pharmacokinetics of buprenorphine. The low limit of detection (<150 pg/mL) permits the analysis of plasma levels of buprenorphine for 24 h after a therapeutic dose of buprenorphine. The drug was extracted from plasma (2–3 mL) with toluene/ 2-butanol at pH 9.4, back-extracted in dilute sulfuric acid, and heated at 110°C. This step led to quantitative loss of methanol followed by ring formation between the 6-methoxy group and the branched side chain of the compound. The derivative was extracted into methylene chloride/2-butanol (pH 9.4) and treated with pentafluoropropionic anhydride. After separation on an OV-1701 capillary column (25 m × 0.3 mm id), buprenorphine (*m/z*: 581-540-497) and norbuprenorphine (*m/z*: 673-658) were detected by MS in SIM mode. After iv injection of buprenorphine in a healthy volunter (0.6 mg), decreasing plasma concentrations of buprenorphine ranged from 7.5 to 0.15 ng/mL. Everhart et al. *(9)* reported difficulties in reproducing the acid-catalyzed degradation of the 7-α side chain published by Blom et al. *(10)*.

In 1989, Ohtani et al. *(11)* found that the SIM acquisition in electron impact mode of detection, even with extensive sample cleanup before derivatization with pentafluoropropionic anhydride, resulted in chromatograms with high background noise, precluding analysis of buprenorphine at subnanogram concentrations in plasma. SIM acquisition of the same derivatized extracts in the positive chemical ionization (PCI) mode of detection increased the sensitivity of the method (LOD of 0.2 ng/mL). The extraction of buprenorphine and its metabolite from plasma was carried out according to the method of Cone et al. *(8)* with minor modifications. Plasma (1 mL) was extracted with ethyl acetate-heptane (4:1 [v/v]) at pH 10.5 after a cleaning extraction step of the specimen with ethyl acetate-heptane (4:1, v/v) at low pH. This organic phase was evaporated and derivatized with toluene-pentafluoropropionic anhydride. GC/MS analysis was performed using an SE-52 Chromosorb W (80–100 mesh, 1 m × 2 mm id) column and isobutane as reactant gas at a chamber pressure of 1 torr (buprenorphine *m/z*: 596-614, norbuprenorphine *m/z*: 688-706). After sl administration of two buprenorphine tablets

(0.1 mg/tablet) to a healthy volunteer, plasma concentrations ranged from 0.5 to 2.4 and from 0.4 to 1.1 ng/mL for buprenorphine and norbuprenorphine, respectively. In two patients with cancer receiving buprenorphine sl tablets or suppositories chronically, plasma concentrations were 0.6 and 1.8 ng/mL for buprenorphine, and 2.0 and 2.9 ng/mL for norbuprenorphine. The method permit to monitor buprenorphine and norbuprenorphine concentrations in clinical practice and pharmacokinetic studies in human.

Kuhlman et al. *(12)* developed a sensitive and specific method capable of measuring both parent buprenorphine and its metabolite, norbuprenorphine, in concentration <1 ng/mL. The method combines the increased sensitivity provided by negative chemical ionization (NCI) with the specificity of tandem mass spectrometry (MS/MS). The solid-phase extraction of plasma (1 mL) was conducted on Clean Screen columns at pH 6.0. After washing with methanol, acetate buffer (pH 4.5), and methanol, the drugs were eluated with methylene chloride-isopropanol-ammonium hydroxide (78:20:2). Heptafluorobutyric (HFB) derivatives of buprenorphine and norbuprenorphine were separated on a DB-5MS capillary column and detected in the NCI mode using ammonia as reagent gas (2 mtorr). Deuterated analog of buprenorphine (d_4) was used for the quantification of the parent drug and norcodeine for its metabolite. Plasma samples obtained from subjects receiving a single 40-mg dose (oral route) or 1- and 2-mg dose (sc) of buprenorphine were analyzed. Table 1 summarizes the results.

The relative response of buprenorphine (LOD: 0.15 ng/mL) in NCI mode was substantially lower than of norbuprenorphine (0.016 ng/mL), certainly owing to the formation of a diderivative by norbuprenorphine rather than formation of a mono-derivative by buprenorphine. This preliminary study was undertaken to investigate buprenorphine pharmacokinetics in six healthy men after iv (1.2 mg), sl (4.0 mg), and buccal (4.0 mg) routes of administration *(13)*.

Moody et al. *(14)* described a sensitive liquid chromatography-electrospray ionization-ms/ms (LC-ESI-MS-MS) method for buprenorphine in human plasma that was compared with a previously validated GC-PCI-MS method. Table 2 reports the comparative observations. Forty plasma samples were tested by both analytical methods. Buprenorphine concentrations in plasma ranged from not detected to 2.1 ng/mL (mean values: 0.1–1.0 ng/mL). Of the two assays described, the LC-ESI-MS-MS method provides the best sensitivity and requires less time to perform (no derivatization step), its major disadvantage being the high cost of the instrumentation. Detection of buprenorphine out to 96 h postdose, or longer, was necessary for accurate determination of pharmacokinetic parameters and to follow the pharmacodynamic effects of the drug.

Table 1
Buprenorphine and Norbuprenorphine Concentrations in Plasma of Patients Receiving Buprenorphine at Different Doses and by Different Routes of Administration

Dose	Buprenorphine	Norbuprenorphine
40 mg (orally)	4.69 ng/mL (peak at 3 h), 0.57 ng/mL at 72 h	3.26 ng/mL (peak at 8 h), 1.32 ng/mL at 48 h
2 mg (subcutaneously)	8.74 ng/mL (peak at 1 h), <0.20 ng/mL at 48 h	0.34 ng/mL (peak at 4 h), 0.12 ng/mL at 48 h
2 mg (subcutaneously)	6.40 ng/mL (30 min), <0.20 ng/mL at 12 h	0.11 ng/mL (30 min), <0.03 ng/mL at 8 h

Table 2
Comparison of LC-ESI-MS-MS and GC-PCI-MS Methods for Determination of Buprenorphine in Human Plasma

	LC-ESI-MS-MS	GC-PCI-MS
Plasma	1 mL	2 mL
Internal standard	Buprenorphine-d_4	Buprenorphine-d_4
Extraction	n-Butyl chloride/acetonitrile (4:1 [v/v]) pH 10.5	n-Butyl chloride/acetonitrile (4:1 [v/v]) pH 10.5
Derivatization	Without	PFPA/toluene
LOQ	0.1 ng/mL	0.5 ng/mL
Positive results[a]	38 (95%)	10 (25%)

[a]Number of positive results for buprenorphine 96 h after sl buprenorphine doses of 2, 8, 16, and 24 mg/kg.

A similar limit of quantitation (LOQ) was achieved with a LC/single-stage MS *(15)* using a more rigorous extraction. Hoja et al. *(16)* developed another analytical procedure for the determination of buprenorphine and its metabolite in hemolyzed whole blood, taking into account the specific problems of postmortem specimens, sometimes hemolyzed. Whole blood first was incubated with *Helix pomatia* extract to hydrolyze the glucuronoconjugated forms followed by a deproteinization with acetonitrile. The clear supernatant was transferred to Extrelut-3 columns, and the drugs were eluated with a mixture of toluene-ether (1:1 [v/v]). Back-extraction was performed in phosphoric acid followed by an ultime extraction with ether at pH 9.0. Chromatographic separation was achieved on a Nucleosil C18 (150 × 1 mm id) reversed-phase column and detection on an API-100 Perkin-Elmer Sciex mass spectrometer equipped with an electrospray-type ionization device. Quantitation limits were 0.1 ng/mL for both parent buprenorphine and its metabolite, norbuprenorphine. Buprenorphine (3.0 ng/mL) and norbuprenorphine (3.1 ng/mL) were found in the postmortem blood of a 24-yr-old Caucasian male drug addict.

Tracqui et al. *(17)* described a simple, rapid (single-step LLE with chloroform/2-propanol/*n*-heptane at pH 8.4), highly sensitive (LOQ of 0.1 and 0.05 ng/mL for buprenorphine and norbuprenorphine, respectively) and specific HPLC/MS method for the determination of buprenorphine and its metabolite in plasma. HPLC separation was performed on a 4-µm NovaPak C18 column (150 × 2.0 mm id) using a continuous flow of 200 µL/min for the mobile phase. A postcolumn split of 1:3 allowed to reduce to 50 µL/min the flow rate infused into the pneumatically assisted electrospray interface. A blood sample obtained from a 23-yr-old male addict under buprenorphine therapy (2.4 mg/day) showed concentrations of 2.7 and 16.9 ng/mL for buprenorphine and norbuprenorphine, respectively. Tracqui et al. *(18)* also adapted the previous procedure to assay buprenorphine and its metabolite in postmortem blood samples. The single-step LLE was replaced by a triple-step LLE starting with chloroform/2-propanol/*n*-heptane at pH 8.4, back-extraction in hydrochloric acid, and finally reextraction with chloroform at pH 8.4. Toxicological investigations in a series of 20 fatalities involving high-dose sl buprenorphine revealed that blood concentrations ranged from 1.1 to 29.0 ng/mL (mean 8.4 ng/mL) and from 0.2 to 12.6 ng/mL (mean 2.6 ng/mL) for buprenorphine and norbuprenorphine, respectively.

To determine indirectly the concentration of conjugated metabolites in a sample, a two-step analysis (with and without hydrolysis) has to be carried out. Recently, Polettini and Huestis *(19)* developed the first method for the simultaneous analysis of buprenorphine, norbuprenorphine, and buprenorphine-glucuronide in plasma. Analytes were isolated from plasma with a C18 SPE column and separated by gradient reversed-phase LC. Detection was achieved on a tandem mass spectrometer equipped with a TurboIonSpray interface. The limit of quantification was established at 0.1 ng/mL for the three analytes. The plasma sample collected 48 h after administration of 12 mg of sl buprenorphine to a volunteer showed buprenorphine, norbuprenorphine, and buprenorphine-glucuronide concentrations of 0.36, 0.33, and 0.41 ng/mL, respectively. Because of its low quantification limit (0.1 ng/mL), the methodology is applicable to the study of buprenorphine and metabolite pharmacokinetics following different routes of drug administration.

3. DETERMINATION OF BUPRENORPHINE IN URINE

Buprenorphine is metabolized in humans primarily by N-dealkylation and conjugation to form norbuprenorphine, which is pharmacologically active, and conjugates of buprenorphine and norbuprenorphine. Buprenorphine has a long plasma half-life. The elimination of the N-desalkyl metabolite is even longer. It is eliminated mainly in the feces (68%), with a small proportion excreted in urine (27%), as metabolite.

The screening method for the identification and semiquantitative determination of buprenorphine in urine published by Hackett et al. *(20)* involves a hydrolysis step with β-glucuronidase (5000 U), a preliminary extraction step with a C18 bonded silica column, an additional purification by TLC, and finally the identification by HPLC. For the extraction, hydrolyzed urine (10 mL at pH 7.5) was deposited on an activated Bond-Elut column and eluated with diethyl ether. The organic phase was evaporated and drugs were deposited on silica gel $60F_{254}$ plates. Buprenorphine was detected by viewing under light at 254 nm and solubilized in methanol. Chromatography was achieved on a 300 × 4 mm id μBondapak C18 column, and the target peak was detected by the uv absorbance at 214 nm. The intermediate TLC step was found to be particularly necessary for the removal of endogenous urine constituents that interfered in the final HPLC analysis. The LOD for the method was approx of 7.5 ng/mL. Several urine samples taken from seven patients who had received treatment for 2 wk with 4 mg of buprenorphine daily (sublingually) showed buprenorphine concentrations ranging from 54 to 260 ng/mL 24 h after the last dose (*n* = 7). For two of them, buprenorphine was detected 72 h afterward with concentrations of 37 and 144 ng/mL. For four other patients of a similar treatment protocol, buprenorphine concentrations were in the range of 21–126 ng/mL 48 h after the last dose (*n* = 4).

The determination of buprenorphine in plasma reported by Martinez et al. *(7)* was adapted for urine specimens. Ten milliliters of urine were hydrolyzed with hydrochloride acid for 1 h at 100°C, before the extraction on Extrelut-20 column at pH 9.2. Instead of diethy ether for plasma, elution was conducted with dichloromethane/2-propanol (85:15 [v/v]). The other analytical parameters remained similar to those used for plasma. Concerning the comparative study (NPD or ECD detection), the same conclusions as for plasma were given for urine samples.

The procedure developed by Schleyer et al. *(6)* for plasma (column-switching solid-phase trace-enrichment HPLC-ECD method) was also applicable to urine specimens without modifications. Results of the validation parameters for urine were closely the same as for plasma. In the urine of patients with sl application, the average buprenorphine concentration was 1.8 ng/mL and 19 ng/mL for norbuprenorphine.

Debrabandere et al. *(21)* proposed a simple, specific, and sensitive screening method for the determination of buprenorphine and norbuprenorphine in urine. Urine (2 mL) was hydrolyzed (β-glucuronidase), extracted with toluene at pH 8.5, back-extracted in hydrochloride acid, and finally reextracted in toluene (pH 8.5). HPLC was carried out on a 5-μm LiChrosorb CN (250 × 4 mm id) column using an acetonitrile-phosphate buffer (pH 3.0) mobile phase (13:87 [v/v]). Electrochemical detection was performed at a potential of 0.75 V and an intensity of 1 nA. LOD was 150 and 250 pg/mg for the metabolite and buprenorphine, respectively. A urine sample collected 10 h after im injection of a single dose of 0.3 mg of buprenorphine revealed an unconjugated buprenorphine concentration of 500 pg/mL and 2 ng/mL for unconjugated norbuprenorphine. The investigators observed that the extracts obtained from deglucuronized urine samples were no longer suitable for analysis with ECD owing to the presence of many coextracting materials.

In another study by Debrabandere et al. *(22)*, this methodology was applied to 50 urine samples obtained from persons suspected of buprenorphine misuse. From the 23 (46%) preselected urine samples (positive radioimmunoassay [RIA] results with a cutoff value of 1 ng/mL), the concentration of unchanged buprenorphine and norbuprenorphine ranged from 0.2 to 15 ng/mL and from 0.6 to 25 ng/mL, respectively. The investigators concluded that HPLC-ECD constituted a valuable alternative method for confirmation of buprenorphine in prescreened urine samples by RIA.

McLinden *(23)* first mentioned buprenorphine as a possible doping agent for greyhounds. Buprenorphine is structurally related to etorphine (known as a doping agent, commercially available as Immobilon or "elephant-juice"), which at very low doses of about 0.1 mg/horse acts as a stimulating agent. It was speculated that a low dose of buprenorphine (0.3 mg/horse) would also induce the specific locomotor activity similar to the response seen with other analgesics, including etorphine, morphine, and fentanyl *(24)*. A ban has been issued by the IOC Medical Commission on the use of buprenorphine together with other narcotic analgesics *(25)*. Debrabandere et al. *(26)* developed confirmatory methods using HPLC-ECD and GC/MS and examined their applicability to postrace equine urine specimens. The GC/MS was developed and validated vs the previously published HPLC-ECD method *(21)*. The new procedure involves enzymatic hydrolysis (β-glucuronidase), LLE (same as for the HPLC-ECD method), and silylation of urine extract. The MS acquisition in SIM mode was able to detect a drug concentration of 100 pg/mL. The unhydrolyzed urine sample collected 1 hour after a single 0.3-mg dose of buprenorphine administered to a horse was positive for buprenorphine (1 ng/mL) and norbuprenorphine (0.4 ng/mL). This GC/MS procedure allows the confirmation of buprenorphine up to 24 h after administration. In a large population of postrace equine urine ($n = 100$), one sample was found to be positive with RIA. HPLC-ECD confirmation was not conclusive but the GC/MS-SIM method revealed the presence of buprenorphine at a concentration of 0.4 ng/mL.

The analytical method published by Cone et al. [8,27] for the determination of buprenorphine and norbuprenorphine started with the hydrolysis of urine samples with β-glucuronidase and sulfatase. Extraction was performed with heptane-ethyl acetate (1:5 [v/v]) at pH 10.0. Drugs were back-extracted in sulfuric acid, washed with hexane, and finally reextracted with heptane/ethyl acetate (1:5 [v/v]) at pH 10.0. The derivatized penta fluoropropionic (PFP) extract was analyzed by GC/ECD or GC/MS-NCI (reagent gas: methane) after separation of the compounds on packed column. Buprenorphine was administered in doses of 1 and 2 mg subcutaneously, 2 and 4 mg sublingually, and 20 and 40 mg orally. The LOD of the assay was approx 10 and 5 ng/mL for buprenorphine and norbuprenorphine, respectively. Absence of free buprenorphine was observed across all doses, routes, and subjects.

Vincent et al. [28] developed an attractive alternative to sophisticated techniques (GC/MS-chemical ionization(CI), LC/MS, or GC-LC/MS/MS) on instruments already available to many laboratories. Hydrolyzed urine was extracted on Bond Elut Certify columns (elution with dichloromethane/isopropyl alcohol, 80:20 [v/v]) and the dry extract derivatized [silylation with N-methyl-N-trimethylsilyltrifluoroacetamide (MSTFA), trimethylchlorosilane (TMCS), (trimethylsilyl)imidazole (TMSIM)]. The analyses were performed on a benchtop mass spectrometer detector operated in EI-SIM mode. The LOD was 0.10 ng/mL for buprenorphine and norbuprenorphine. Data obtained from five patients undergoing buprenorphine therapy showed total parent and metabolite concentrations ranging from 1007 to 3316 and from 636 to 6990 ng/mg of creatinine, respectively.

The procedure to test buprenorphine and its metabolite in postmortem blood samples published by Tracqui et al. [18] was also used to assay urine specimens. The triple-step LLE followed by the HPLC-IS-MS technique was able to detect the drug in a series of 20 fatalities involving high-dose sl buprenorphine when the sample was available. Urine concentrations ranged from 4.0 to 1033 ng/mL ($n = 14$) and from 6.6 to 230 ng/mL ($n = 14$) for buprenorphine and norbuprenorphine, respectively. The performance of the method for urine was the same as that described for blood samples.

4. DETERMINATION OF BUPRENORPHINE IN BIOLOGICAL TISSUES

The studies of Cone et al. *(8,27)* and Tracqui et al. *(18)* reported the determination of buprenorphine in unusual biological specimens such as feces, bile, gastric content or tissues (liver, brain, kidney, and myocardium). In the reports of Cone et al. *(8,27)*, feces samples were homogenized in methanol, and the supernatant was extracted as for urine after decantation and evaporation. The excretion of buprenorphine and norbuprenorphine was investigated in feces for two individual subjects following 10-, 20-, and 40-mg oral doses of buprenorphine. Free and conjugated buprenorphine were present in all samples, with free buprenorphine exceeding that of the conjugated metabolite. Norbuprenorphine was present in all but one sample tested, with free metabolite content exceeding the conjugated form. The greatest amount of drug and metabolite eliminated in feces occurred at 4–6 d following administration of buprenorphine, at times when there was very little urinary excretion of conjugated buprenorphine.

In the study by Tracqui et al. *(18)*, tissue samples were obtained from autopsy cases. Specimens were first homogenized in water and then extracted like other biological fluids. Toxicological investigations showed that buprenorphine concentration in tissues was markely higher than blood level whatever the dose and route of administration. This was owing to an almost complete drug distribution to the extravascular compartments. High concentrations of both buprenorphine and its metabolite were also observed in bile (575–72,650 ng/mL for buprenorphine and 41 to >30,000 ng/mL for norbuprenorphine), as a consequence of the massive biliary excretion of the drug.

Finally, identification and quantification of buprenorphine in sweat was proposed by Kintz et al. *(29)*. Sweat patches were applied for 5 d on 16 heroin addicts under buprenorphine substitution maintenance (0.4–6.0 mg/day). The target drugs were extracted from the absorbent pad using methanol in the presence of deuterated internal standard. The extract was directly analyzed by the HPLC-MS system previously described *(17)*. With an LOD of 0.2 ng/patch, buprenorphine was detectable in all sweat patches. Concentrations ranged from 1.3 to 153.2 ng/patch. Norbuprenorphine was detected in only one case (3.1 ng/patch). This new technology was proposed for the treatment and monitoring of substance abusers.

5. DETERMINATION OF BUPRENORPHINE IN HAIR

Information about recent exposure to a drug acquired by blood and urine analyses can be complemented by hair analysis, which can provide a retrospective view of drug intake over several weeks or months, depending on the length of the analyzed strand (each centimeter corresponds to approx 1 mo).

Kintz (30) published the first report concerning the determination of buprenorphine in hair. Hair was decontaminated, pulverized, and incubated overnight at 56°C in 0.1 N HCl. After neutralization, the homogenate was extracted according to the procedure published by Debrabandere et al. (21) for determination of buprenorphine in urine. Buprenorphine and its dealkylated metabolite, norbuprenorphine, were separated on a 5-μm Lichrosorb CN column (250 × 4 mm) using a 10 mM phosphate buffer (pH 4.0)-acetonitrile-1-heptane sulfonic acid-butylamine (85:17:2:0.01 [v/v]) mobile phase at a flow rate of 1 mL/min. Coulometric detection was achieved with a first electrode potential value at +0.15 V and a second electrode at +0.50 V. The detection limits were 0.01 and 0.02 ng/mg for buprenorphine and norbuprenorphine, respectively. In three buprenorphine addicts admitted to a detoxification program and reporting daily use, buprenorphine concentrations in hair were 0.48, 0.50, and 0.59 ng/mg. As is generally the case for drugs, the concentrations of the metabolite were lower (0.06, 0.15, and 0.14 ng/mg).

The same procedure was applied to 14 heroin addicts admitted for 2 or 3 mo to a detoxification center (31). Hair samples were screened by RIA and confirmed by HPLC-coulometric detection and GLC-MS. GC was achieved using the method of Blom and Bondesson (10). LC was evaluated using two different interfaces: a particle beam and an electrospray. With RIA, all the hair samples obtained from the treated subjects contained buprenorphine with concentrations ranging from 0.01 to 0.47 ng/mg. Both LC and GC mass spectrometry procedures were not sensitive enough to detect buprenorphine in hair. Limits of detection were 10, 5, and 0.5 ng/mg with LC/particle beam, LC/electrospray, and GC/MS, respectively, and 40 pg/mg by RIA. It was demonstrated that buprenorphine was thermally unstable in the heated source of the mass spectrometer. The thermal degradation can be avoided by chemical modification, which involves the ring formation between the side chain and the methoxy group. HPLC coupled to coulometric detection was able to detect buprenorphine in all 14 hair samples, with concentrations ranging from 0.02 to 0.59 ng/mg. Norbuprenorphine was detected with concentrations ranging from not detected to 0.15 ng/mg ($n = 11$). Buprenorphine was generally present in hair at concentrations approx 2 to 18 times higher than norbuprenorphine concentrations. Although the limited subject data preclude generalization, the obtained results suggested that a dose-response relationship exists.

Tracqui et al. (17) measured buprenorphine and norbuprenorphine by HPLC/MS after acid hydrolysis (0.1 N HCl, overnight at 56°C) in the presence of a deuterated analog of the parent drug. The homogenate was extracted using chloroform/2-propanol/n-heptane (25:10:65 [v/v]) at pH 8.4. Separation was obtained on a 4-μm Novapak C18 column (150 × 2 mm id) using a gradient of 2 mM NH$_4$COOH buffer/acetonitrile mobile phase at a flow rate of 200 μL/min. After a postcolumn split (1:3), analytes were infused in a mass analyzer equipped with an ion-spray interface. The concentrations determined in the hair of six addicts under substitutive therapy with buprenorphine ranged from 4 to 140 pg/mg, with a detection limit of 4 pg/mg and from not detected to 67 pg/mg with a detection limit of 2 pg/mg, for buprenorphine and norbuprenorphine, respectively. In another study by Tracqui et al. *(18)*, the two compounds were solubilized the same way and isolated after a triple-step extraction procedure detailed before. In 11 hair specimens obtained from 20 fatalities, buprenorphine concentrations ranged from not detected to 597 pg/mg, whereas norbuprenorphine was never detected.

In 1999, Vincent et al. *(28)* developed an analytical procedure for determination of buprenorphine and norbuprenorphine in both urine and hair samples that differs only by the pretreatment step. The hydrolysis step used for hair was the acidic incubation proposed by Kintz *(30)*. The LOD and quantification were 2 and 5 pg/mg for each compound, respectively. For five patients in a substitution treatment program, the measured concentrations of buprenorphine and norbuprenorphine in hair ranged from 6 to 361 and 29 to 785 pg/mg, respectively. The investigators observed that norbuprenorphine was often found in higher concentration than the parent drug. They noted that this result was somewhat unusual but in accordance with the findings of Valdez et al. *(32)*. They concluded that norbuprenorphine appeared to be more incorporated in hair than the parent compound. The same conclusions were reported by Wilkins et al. *(33)* for four subjects maintained on the assigned doses for 4 wk and increased doses at 4-wk intervals for up to 16 wk. Table 3 provides the concentrations of several hair segments determined by LC/MS/MS.

In another study published by Wilkens et al. *(34)*, 12 subjects received 8 mg of sl buprenorphine for a maximum of 180 d. Hair strands were collected after the treatment period and stored at –20°C. For the analysis, hair samples were digested overnight in 1 N NaOH in the presence of deuterated internal standards (buprenorphine- and norbuprenorphine-d$_4$). The digests were extracted using n-butyl chloride/acetonitrile (4:1 [v/v]) at pH 10.5 in the presence of sodium bicarbonate buffer. Separation was obtained on a C8 Solvent Miser column (2.1 × 150 mm) with an isocratic mobile phase of water/methanol/acetonitrile (25:30:45) containing 1% formic acid. Detection was achieved using MS/MS. The two target compounds were detected in 11 of the 12 subjects, with concentrations ranging from 3.1 to 123.8 and from 4.8 to 1517.8 pg/mg for buprenorphine and norbuprenorphine, respectively. With one

Table 3
Buprenorphine and Norbuprenorphine in Several Hair Segments of Subjects Maintained on Assigned Doses for 4 wk and Increased Doses at 4 wk Intervals for Up to 16 wk.

Subject	Buprenorphine (pg/mg)	Norbuprenorphine (pg/mg)
A	4.5–45.5	4.8–54.5
B	5.3–16.1	20.8–153.4
C	17.8–113.6	67.7–884.0
D	8.1–156.8	43.7–1438.5

exception, norbuprenorphine was always present in higher concentrations in hair segments than was the parent compound (ratio of at least 1:3).

Recently, Cirimele et al. *(35)* investigated complementary experimentations in order to explain the contradictory observations of buprenorphine-to-norbuprenorphine ratio in hair. Thirty-three hair specimens were obtained from drug addicts and assayed for buprenorphine using HPLC/MS. Hair strands (approx 100 mg) were twice decontaminated in 5 mL of methylene chloride for 2 min at room temperature. After pulverization, 50 mg of powdered hair was incubated in 0.1 N HCl, overnight at 56°C, in the presence of each deuterated analog of buprenorphine (buprenorphine-d_4) and norbuprenorphine (norbuprenorphine-d_3). After neutralization, the solubilization medium was extracted using chloroform/2-propanol/n-heptane (25:10:65 [v/v]) at pH 8.4. Analyses were performed by HPLC/MS as described before *(18)*. Figure 1 shows the typical chromatogram of a hair extract. Buprenorphine (*m/z*: 468–414) and norbuprenorphine (*m/z*: 414) concentrations were 521 and 150 pg/mg, respectively. Figures 2 (buprenorphine) and 3 (norbuprenorphine) show the mass spectra of both compounds.

The decontamination washes were also analyzed using the same purification procedure. LOQ was 0.01 ng/mg for the two target compounds. About the 33 hair specimens were tested, buprenorphine was detected in higher concentrations than norbuprenorphine in 14 cases, but in 16 cases the metabolite was predominant (same concentration in 3 cases). Buprenorphine concentrations ranged from not detected to 1.19 ng/mg and from not detected to 1.21 ng/mg for norbuprenorphine. For the 66 analyzed washes, buprenorphine was present in higher quantity than its metabolite in 40 cases, and norbuprenorphine was predominant in only 7 cases. In 19 cases, the target compounds were not detected. The investigators concluded that the decontamination procedure with methylene chloride affects the drug content of hair. Buprenorphine was preferentially and quantitatively lost during this first step of the wash procedure.

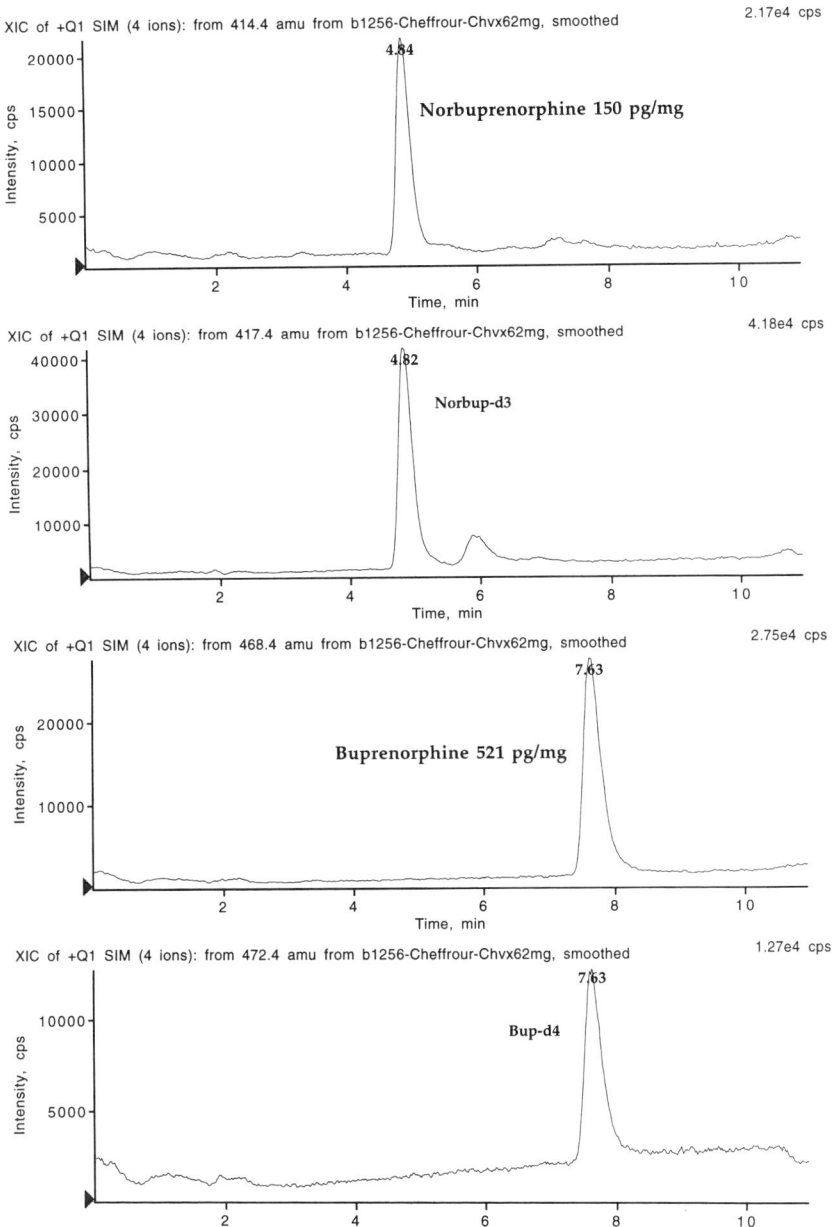

Fig. 1 Reconstructed chromatogram of hair specimen positive for buprenorphine (521 pg/mg) and norbuprenorphine (150 pg/mg). The deuterated analogs of each compound were used for the quantification.

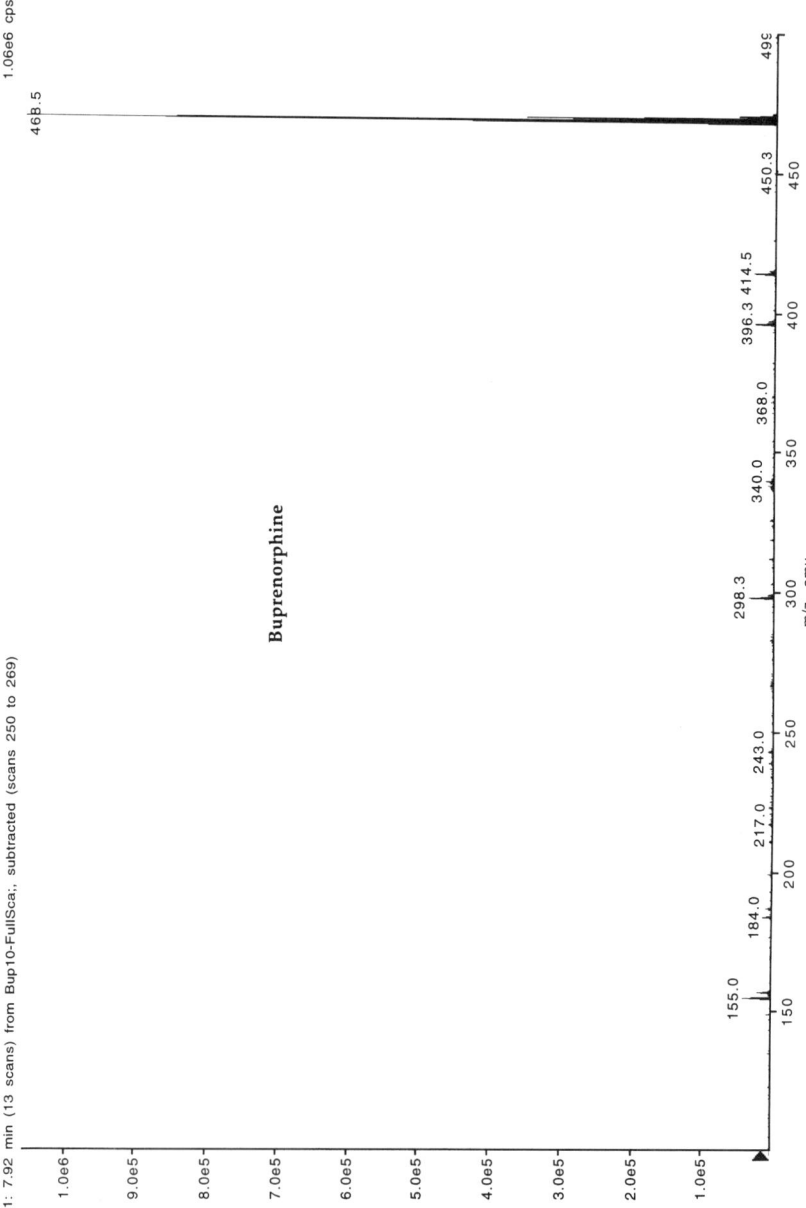

Fig. 2 Mass spectra of buprenorphine (m/z 100–500) obtained by HPLC-ion-spray-ms.

Techniques for Determination of Buprenorphine

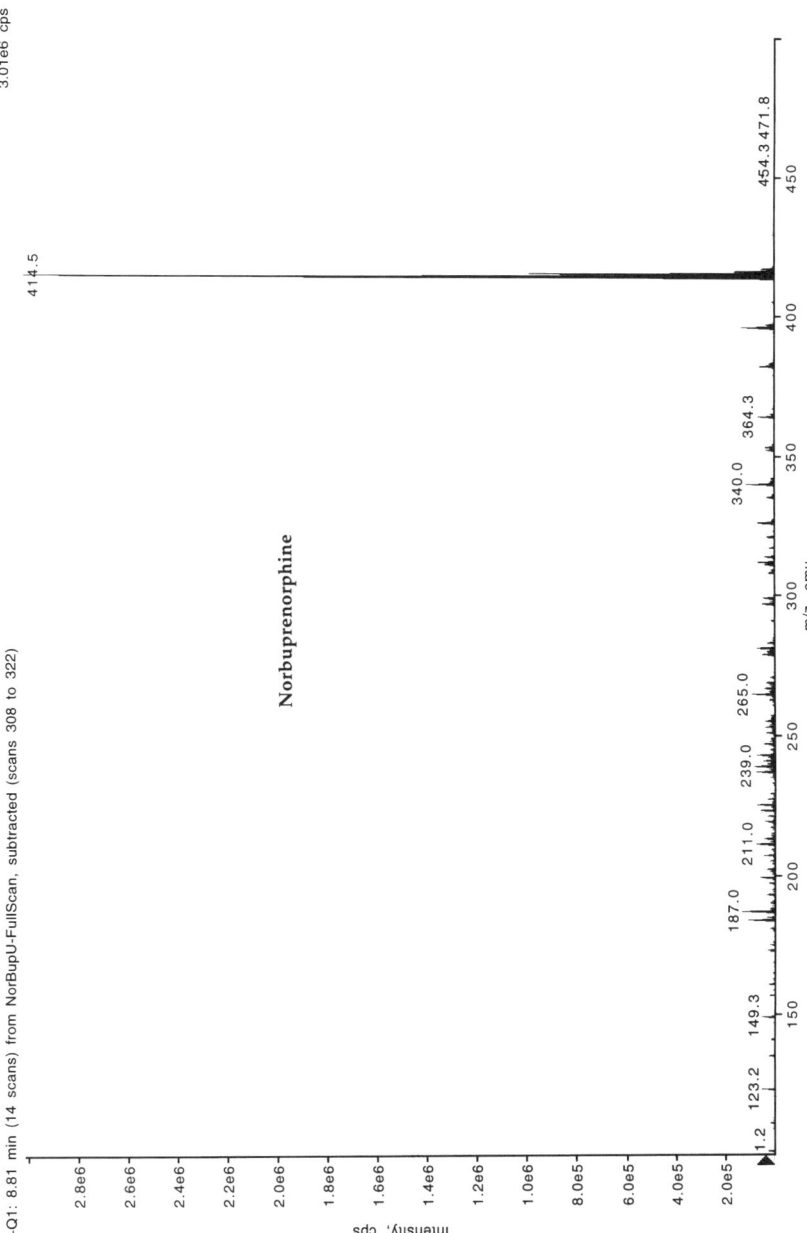

Fig. 3 Mass spectra of norbuprenorphine (m/z 100–500) obtained by HPLC-ion-spray-ms.

6. CONCLUSION

The literature on the analytical chemistry of buprenorphine and norbuprenorphine is rich, with methods based on HPLC or GC coupled with numerous detectors. HPLC, with the exeption of the recently published HPLC/MS methods, does not appear to possess the routine sensitivity required for the reliable measurement of buprenorphine in plasma. GC/MS requires long, complex, and tedious extraction procedures (for an extensive sample cleanup) before the derivatization step. At this time, HPLC-ion spray-MS and HPLC-ion spray-MS/MS represent the state of the art in terms of specificity and sensibility.

REFERENCES

1. Lloyd-Jones JG, Robinson P, Henson R, Biggs SR, Taylor T. Plasma concentration and disposition of buprenorphine after intravenous and intramuscular doses to baboons. Eur J Drug Metab Pharmacokinet 1980;5:233–9.
2. Tebbett IR. Analysis of buprenorphine by high-performance liquid chromatography. J Chromatogr 1985;347:411–3.
3. Lagrange F, Pehourcq F, Baumevieille M, Begaud B. Determination of buprenorphine in plasma by liquid chromatography: application to heroin-dependent subjects. J Pharm Biomed Anal, 1998;16:1295–300.
4. Garrett ER, Chandran VR. Pharmacokinetics of morphine and its surrogates VI: bioanalysis, solvolysis kinetics, solubility, pka values, and protein binding of buprenorphine, J Pharm Sci 1985;74: 515–24.
5. Ho S-T, Wang J-J, Ho W. Determination of buprenorphine by high-performance liquid chromatography with fluorescence detection: application to human and rabbit pharmacokinetic studies. J Chromatogr 1991;570:339–50.
6. Schleyer E, Lohmann R, Rolf C, Gralow A, Kaufmann CC, Unterhalt M, Hiddemann W. Column-switching solid-phase trace-enrichment HPLC method for measurement of buprenorphine and norbuprenorphine in human plasma and urine by electrochemical detection. J Chromatogr 1993;614:275–83.
7. Martinez D, Jurado MC, Repetto M. Analysis of buprenorphine in plasma and urine by gas chromatography. J Chromatogr 1990;528: 459–63.
8. Cone EJ, Gorodetzky CW, Yousefnejad D, Darwin WD. ^{63}Ni electron-capture gas-chromatography assay for buprenorphine and metabolites in human urine and feces. J Chromatogr 1985;337:291–300.
9. Everhart ET, Cheung P, Shwonek P, Zabel K, Tisdale EC, Jacob III P, Mendelson J, Jones RT. Subnanogram-concentration measurement of buprenorphine in human plasma by electron-capture capillary gas chromatography: application to pharmacokinetics of sublingual buprenorphine. Clin Chem 1997;43:2292–302.
10. Blom Y, Bondesson U. Analysis of buprenorphine and its N-dealkylated metabolite in plasma and urine by selected-ion monitoring. J Chrom 1985;338:89–98.

11. Ohtani M, Shibuya F, Kotaki H, Uchino K, Saitoh Y, Nakagawa F, Quantitative determination of buprenorphine and its active metabolite, norbuprenorphine, in human plasma by gas chromatography-chemical ionization mass spectrometry. J Chrom 1989;487:469–75.
12. Kuhlman JJ, Magluilo J, Cone E, Levine B. Simultaneous assay of buprenorphine and norbuprenorphine by negative chemical ionization tandem mass spectrometry. J Anal Toxicol 1996;20:229–35.
13. Kuhlman JJ, Lalani S, Magluilo J, Levine B, Darwin WD, Johnson RE, Cone EJ. Human pharmacokinetics of intravenous, sublingual, and buccal buprenorphine. J Anal Toxicol 1996;20:369–78.
14. Moody DE, Laycock JD, Spanbauer AC, Crouch DJ, Foltz RL, Josephs JL, Amass L, Bickel WK. Determination of buprenorphine in human plasma by gas chromatography-positive ion chemical ionozation mass spectrometry and liquid chromatography-tandem mass spectrometry. J Anal Toxicol, 1997;21:406–14.
15. Hoja H, Marquet P, Verneuil B, Lotfi H, Dupuy JL, Dreyfuss MF, Lachâtre G. Dosage de buprénorphine et de norbuprénorphine dans l'urine et le sérum par chromatographie liquide couplée à la spectrométrie de masse avec ionisation de type "électrospray" (LC/ES/MS), Analusis, 1996;24:104–7.
16. Hoja H, Marquet P, Verneuil B, Lotfi H, Dupuy JL, Lachâtre G. Determination of buprenorphine and norbuprenorphine in whole blood by liquid chromatography-mass spectrometry. J Anal Toxicol 1997;21:160–5.
17. Tracqui A, Kintz P, Mangin P. HPLC/MS determination of buprenorphine and norbuprenorphine in biological fluids and hair samples. J Forensic Sci 1997;42:111–4.
18. Tracqui A, Kintz P, Ludes B. Buprenorphine-related deaths among drug addicts in France: A report on 20 fatalities, J Anal Toxicol 1998;22:430–4.
19. Polettini A, Huestis MA. Simultaneous determination of buprenorphine, norbuprenorphine, and buprenorphine-glucuronide in plasma by liquid chromatography-tandem mass spectrometry. J Chrom B 2001;754:447–59.
20. Hackett LP, Dusci LJ, Ilett KF, Seow SSW, Quigley AJ. Sensitive screening method for buprenorphine in urine. J Chrom 1986;374:400–4.
21. Debrabandere L, Van Boven M, Daenens P. High-performance liquid chromatography with electrochemical detection of buprenorphine and its major metabolite in urine. J Chrom 1991;564: 557–66.
22. Debrabandere L, Van Boven M, Daenens P. Analysis of buprenorphine in urine specimens. J Forensic Sci 1992;37:82–9.
23. McLinden VF. In: Dunnett N, Kimber KJ, eds., Proceedings of the 21st international meeting, The International Association of Forensic Toxicologists, Brighton:1984.
24. Combie J, Shults T, Tobin T. In: Proceedings of the 3rd international symposium on equine medication, Tobin T, Blake JW, Woods WE, eds., Lexington, KY:1979.
25. Dirix A, Knuttgen HG, Tittel K. eds., The olympic book of sports medicine, vol. 1, Blackwell, Oxford:1988.
26. Debrabandere L, Van Boven M, Laruelle L, Daenens P. Routine detection of buprenorphine in horse urine: possibilities and limitations of the combined use of radioimmunoassay, liquid chromatography and gas chromatography-mass spectrometry. Anal Chimica Acta 1993;275:295–303.

27. Cone EJ, Gorodetzky CW, Yousefnejad D, Buchwald WF, Johnson RE. The metabolisme and excretion of buprenorphine in humans. Drug Metab Dispos 1984; 12:577–81.
28. Vincent F, Bessard J, Vacheron J, Mallaret M, Bessard G. Determination of buprenorphine and norbuprenorphine in urine and hair by gas chromatography-mass spectrometry. J Anal Toxicol 1999;23:270–9.
29. Kintz P, Tracqui A, Mangin P, Edel Y. Sweat testing in opioid users with a sweat patch. J Anal Toxicol 1996;20:393–7.
30. Kintz P. Determination of buprenorphine and its dealkylated metabolite in human hair. J Anal Toxicol 1993;17:443–4.
31. Kintz P, Cirimele V, Edel Y, Jamey C, Mangin P. Hair analysis for buprenorphine and its dealkylated metabolite by radioimmunoassay and confirmation by LC-ECD. J Forensic Sci 1994;39:1497–503.
32. Valdez AS, Wilkins DG, Slawson MH, Sison C, Ling W, Rollins DE. Buprenorphine and norbuprenorphine in human hair of substance abuse treatment subjects. Poster presented in College on Problems of Drug Dependence, 60th annual scientific meeting, Scottsdale, AZ, 1998.
33. Wilkins D, Slawson M, Valdez A, Sison C, Huber A, Ling W, Rollins D. Buprenorphine, norbuprenorphine and melanin in human hair. In: Proceedings of the SOFT-TIAFT joint meeting, Albuquerque, NM, 1998.
34. Wilkins DG, Rollins DE, Valdez AS, Mizuno A, Krueger GG, Cone E.J. A retrospective study of buprenorphine and norbuprenorphine in human hair after multiples doses. J Anal Toxicol 1999;23:409–15.
35. Cirimele V, Kintz P, Lohner S, Ludes B. Buprenorphine to norbuprenorphine ratio in human hair. J Anal Toxicol 2000;24:448-9.

Chapter 8

Buprenorphine-Related Deaths

Pascal Kintz

1. INTRODUCTION

Buprenorphine is a semisynthetic opioid derivative, closely related to morphine, that is obtained from thebaine after a seven-step chemical procedure. At low doses (typically 0.3–0.6 mg intravenously or intramuscularly), buprenorphine is a powerful analgesic, 25–40 times more potent than morphine, with mixed agonist/antagonist activity on central receptors *(1)*.

Under the tradename Temgesic® at dosages of 0.2 mg, buprenorphine has been widely prescribed for about 20 yr for the treatment of moderate to severe pain as well as in anesthesiology for premedication or anesthetic induction. More recently, it has also been recognized as a medication of interest for the substitutive management of opiate-dependent individuals. Under the tradename Subutex®, a high-dosage formulation (0.4-, 2-, and 8-mg tablets for sublingual use) has beenavailable in France since February 1996 in this specific indication. Contrary to methadone, which is delivered on a daily basis in specific centers and continuous survey of the patient by urine analysis is achieved each week, Subutex may be ordered by any physician up to 28 d and is supplied by any pharmacist. Patients are not required to take the drug in the presence of the physician or pharmacist. Today, this drug is largely used in France for the treatment of about 60,000–80,000 heroin addicts, but it can also be easily found on the black market.

Since the first fatality observed by Tracqui et al. *(2)* in August 1996, several cases have been recorded by French toxicologists. In 1998, Tracqui et al. *(3)* reported on data of 20 fatalities collected from five French laboratories. In all cases but one, a concomitant intake of psychotropics (mostly benzodiazepines) was observed. More recently, an article presented the results of a new retrospective survey on buprenorphine-related deaths in the region of

From *Forensic Science and Medicine: Buprenorphine Therapy of Opiate Addiction*
Edited by: P. Kintz and P. Marquet © Humana Press Inc., Totowa, NJ

Strasbourg from March 1998 to July 2000 and from 13 different forensic centers in France from mid-1996 to March 2000 *(4)*.

Besides other sources of information (such as drug enforcement services, customs, intensive care units), the epidemiological data collected from forensic toxicologists may be of value to follow the evolution of narcotic deaths over the course of time. Each year, in addition to the records of the forensic toxicologists, an official record of deaths from overdose of buprenorphine is computed by a centralized French agency (Office pour la Repression du Trafic Illicite des Stupéfiants). By cross-comparing these two independant sources of information, it clearly appears that the total number of buprenorphine-related deaths is largely underestimated by the official statistics, leading to a false conclusion that buprenorphine is a safe alternative to methadone *(5)*.

2. FORENSIC ASPECTS

In all cases, autopsies revealed signs of asphyxia (e.gh., cyanosis, multivisceral congestion, pulmonary edema) but showed no signs of violence. No other cause of death could be established by experienced pathologists.

In Strasbourg, buprenorphine and norbuprenorphine were assayed in postmortem blood by using an high-performance liquid chromatography/mass spectrometry (MS) procedure *(6)*. Other centers used either gas chromatography (GC)/MS (3 laboratories) or liquid chromatography (LC)/MS (10 laboratories) to test for buprenorphine, according to their own validated procedure *(7,8)*.

In addition to specific analysis of buprenorphine, a complementary screening of the postmortem blood was performed in all subjects using immunoassays (fluorescene-polarization immunossay or enzyme-multiplied immunossay technique), ultraviolet spectrophotometry (carbon monoxide), GC/FID (meprobamate, ethanol), head-space GC/nitrogen-phosphorus detectors (NPD) or colorimetry (cyanides), head-space GC/flame ionization detection (FID) or -MS (usual organic solvents) and LC/diode array detection (DAD) + GLC/MS (pharmaceuticals, drugs of abuse).

3. BUPRENORPHINE FATALITIES

Generally, when interpreting a blood concentration from a postmortem case, the toxicologist can find helpful information in databases presenting therapeutic, toxic, and lethal concentrations. Unfortunately, there are no suitable references in the literature, for buprenorphine. At best, therapeutic concentrations can be evaluated from clinical studies in the range of 2–20 ng/mL *(9)*. No toxic nor lethal concentrations are available, because only French authors have reported deaths involving buprenorphine. Consequently Tracqui et al.

(3) attributed 20 fatalities to buprenorphine poisoning, even at therapeutic concentrations, since no other cause of death was obvious (Table 1). They concluded that buprenorphine can be life-threatening without overdosage, when associated with psychotropic drugs.

Recent results, collected both in Strasbourg and in several other centers, confirm these preliminary findings *(4)*. Toxicological data are reported in Tables 2 and 3. Blood levels for buprenorphine ranged from 0.1 to 76.0 ng/mL (mean: 9.8 ng/mL) and for norbuprenorphine ranged from 0.1 to 65.0 ng/mL (mean: 7.6 ng/mL).

Of these 137 subjects (Tables 1–3), 115 were male (84%), most of them with a low socioprofessional status. Circumstances of death were strongly suggestive of a drug fatality in about two-thirds of subjects: empty packages of Subutex and/or remains of buprenorphine (e.g., in spoons or straws), other psychotropics (pharmaceuticals or drugs of abuse) or used syringes. Evidence of violence was never found at autopsy, but all corpses presented the features of a prolonged asphyxiation (deep cyanosis, multivisceral congestion, pulmonary edema). These signs are very usual in all deaths involving central nervous system (CNS) depressants, especially in opiate-related fatalities. Needle marks suggesting recent iv injections were observed in about half of the subjects. Eight typical cases, observed in Strasbourg, are detailed Table 4. In addition to these 137 cases, 2 other cases were observed, which were classified as suicide, with buprenorphine blood concentrations of 144 and 3276 ng/mL *(10)*.

Buprenorphine was detected in 33 of the 37 hair samples assayed in Strasbourg, showing a chronic use of the drug for the individuals concerned. Concentrations ranged from 6 to 1080, and not detected to 1020 pg/mg for buprenorphine and norbuprenorphine, respectively.

Whatever the dose and route of administration, buprenorphine distributes almost completely to the extravascular compartments with the predictable consequence of tissue concentrations being markedly higher than blood levels (Table 5). From the data of Tracqui et al. *(3)* demonstrate that buprenorphine sequestration occurred in the kidney, brain, and liver. Regarding norbuprenorphine, the metabolite was generally undetectable in the myocardium and in the brain. The latter result is consistent with experimental studies in which virtually no norbuprenorphine was shown to cross the blood-brain barrier *(11)*. However, in a case of massive overdose, Gaulier et al. *(10)* were able to identify norbuprenorphine in the decedent's brain.

High concentrations of both buprenorphine and norbuprenorphine were observed in the bile. For buprenorphine, the average bile/blood ratio was about 10,000. These outstanding discrepancies between blood and bile are a consequence of the massive biliary excretion of buprenorphine and metabolites.

Table 1
Toxicological Data in the First 20 Fatalities Observed in France[a]

Buprenorphine concentrations in blood	1.1–29.0 ng/mL, mean: 8.4 ng/mL
Norbuprenorphine concentrations in blood	0.2–12.6 ng/mL, mean: 2.6 ng/mL
Buprenorphine + EtOH + various	6 cases (30%)
Buprenorphine + benzodiazepines	18 cases (90%)
Buprenorphine + neuroleptics	3 cases (15%)
Buprenorphine + other psychotropics	3 cases (15%)
Buprenorphine + narcotics	4 cases (20%)
Buprenorphine + cocaine	0 cases

[a]Adapted from ref. 3.

Table 2
Toxicological Data in 39 Fatalities Observed in Strasbourg[a]

Buprenorphine concentrations in blood	0.5–51.0 ng/mL, mean: 10.2 ng/mL
Norbuprenorphine concentrations in blood	0.2–47.1 ng/mL, mean: 8.2 ng/mL
Buprenorphine + EtOH + various	10 cases (25.6%)
Buprenorphine + benzodiazepines	31 cases (79.5%)
Buprenorphine + neuroleptics	18 cases (46.2%)
Buprenorphine + other psychotropics	8 cases (20.5%)
Buprenorphine + narcotics	3 cases (7.6%)
Buprenorphine + cocaine	0 cases
Buprenorphine + cannabis	22 cases (56.4%)

[a]Adapted from ref. 4.

Table 3
Toxicological Data in 78 Fatalities Observed in 13 French Centers[a]

Buprenorphine concentrations in blood	0.1–76.0 ng/mL, mean: 12.6 ng/mL
Norbuprenorphine concentrations in blood[b]	<0.1–65.0 ng/mL, mean: 10.6 ng/mL
Buprenorphine + EtOH + various	24 cases (30.8%)
Buprenorphine + benzodiazepines	60 cases (76.9%)
Buprenorphine + neuroleptics	19 cases (24.3%)
Buprenorphine + other psychotropics	16 cases (20.5%)
Buprenorphine + narcotics	20 cases (25.6%)
Buprenorphine + cocaine	6 cases (7.7%)
Buprenorphine + cannabis	36 cases (46.2%)

[a]Adapted from ref. 4.
[b]Norbuprenorphine was measured in only 61 cases.

Table 4
Eight Typical Fatalities Observed in Strasbourg

Case	Buprenorphine in blood (ng/mL)	Norbuprenorphine in blood (ng/mL)	Other compounds in blood
Woman, 21 yr-old, found in her bed, needle marks	3.3	1.4	Bromazepam: 304 ng/mL, nordiazepam: 1060 ng/mL, ethanol: 0.18 g/L
Man, 32 yr-old, found at home, needle marks	13.4	6.8	Amisulpride: 1.04 mg/L, meprobamate: 55.3 mg/L, levomepromazine: 157 ng/mL, clobazam: 469 ng/mL, tropatepine: 206 ng/mL
Man, 32 yr-old, found at home of friend, under substitution	3.7	1.5	Bromazepam: 106 ng/mL, nordiazepam: 1510 ng/mL, cyamemazine: 314 ng/mL
Man, 27 yr-old, found in garage, under substitution	4.9	2.6	Ethanol: 0.85 g/L, 7-aminoflunitrazepam: 43 ng/mL
Man, 22 yr-old, found in street, homeless, under substitution	2.6	1.8	Nordiazepam: 6540 ng/mL, meprobamate: 83 mg/L, THC-COOH: 0.9 ng/mL
Man, 19 yr-old, found dead after party, polydrug abuser	1.8	0.6	Ethanol: 0.34 g/L, MDMA: 157 ng/mL, THC: 1.3 ng/mL
Woman, 30 yr-old, found at home, no prescription of Subutex	7.5	14.9	Nordiazepam: 5020 ng/mL, 7-aminoflunitrazepam: 56 ng/mL
Man, 28 yr-old, known to be opiate opiate addict, needle marks	8.7	5.3	Fluoxetine: 301 ng/mL, cyamemazine: 421 ng/mL, ethanol: 0.32 g/L 7-aminoflunitrazepam: 96 ng/mL

Table 5
Distribution of Buprenorphine and Norbuprenorphine in Tissues[a]

Tissue	Buprenorphine	Norbuprenorphine[b]
Bile ($n = 13$)	577–72,640 ng/mL	41 to >30,000 ng/mL
Liver ($n = 8$)	4–273 ng/g	ND to 64 ng/g, 7 (+) cases
Brain ($n = 6$)	7–151 ng/g	ND to 6 ng/g, 1 (+) case
Kidney ($n = 7$)	8–138 ng/g	ND to 24 ng/g, 4 (+) cases
Myocardium ($n = 6$)	3–12 ng/g	ND to 4 ng/g, 2 (+) cases

[a]Adapted from ref. 3.
[b]ND; not détected.

Bile, therefore, appears as the sample of choice for the systematic screening for buprenorphine.

Fatalities involving buprenorphine alone seem highly unusual: all cases but two involved a concomitant intake of psychotropics. In these cases, the cause of death was listed as tracheobronchial inhalation (Mendelsson syndrome). The blood buprenorphine concentrations were 0.8 and 3.1 ng/mL.

In a case from 1979, Banks (12) reported the ingestion of a large dose (35–40 tablets of 0.4 mg each) of buprenorphine with a suicidal intent in which symptoms were minimal and recovery complete.

Benzodiazepines ranked first in association, since they were present in 109 deaths (of which 79 with nordiazepam). The role of associated benzodiazepines had been previously emphasized in several clinical reports of severe, nonfatal respiratory depression observed when giving buprenorphine to anesthetized patients (13). It is suggested that the CNS depressant effects of buprenorphine may be synergically potentialized by some benzodiazepines (otherwise almost harmless if taken alone). Kilicarslan and Sellers (14) recently demonstrated a lack of interaction between buprenorphine and flunitrazepam metabolism. In 1999, Clément et al. (15) pointed out the potential risk of death when buprenorphine is administered along with benzodiazepines.

Similar interactions probably exist between buprenorphine and other psychotropics, such as neuroleptics and antidepressants. Among the neuroleptics (40 cases), cyamemazine was present in 28 cases. Antidepressants (20 cases) were tricyclic (9 cases) or serotonin reuptake inhibitors (11 cases).

A concomitant intake of other narcotics was observed in 27 cases, mostly outside the region of Strasbourg. These narcotics included morphine (15 cases with 8 at toxic concentrations), codeine (2 cases), methadone (4 cases), pethidine (1 case), and propoxyphene (5 cases).

A fatal association involving ethanol and buprenorphine, without any other drug, was observed in 4 cases, at the following concentrations : 0.8 and 2.18, 1.3 and 0.73, 11.4 and 0.4, and 18.0 ng/mL and 2.29 g/L for buprenorphine and ethanol, respectively. Although not yet described for buprenorphine, a pharmacokinetic interaction between heroin and ethanol has been observed in heroin-related deaths *(16)*.

Injecting buprenorphine intravenously after crushing the sublingual tablets probably constitutes another risk factor of potential fatal overdosage. Most of the clinical reports on buprenorphine-induced respiratory depression concern iv administration *(17)*. This route of administration involves a quasi-instantaneous saturation of the central opiate receptors and a maximization of buprenorphine bioavailability, which is otherwise poor, especially only 20–30%. According to Pinoit et al. *(18)*, the combination of buprenorphine injection intravenously with benzodiazepines can be compared for addicts, in terms of pharmacological effects, to heroin abuse. Substantial risk of injecting misuse is associated with large-scale diffusion of buprenorphine for drug maintenance treatment. Therefore, Obadia et al. *(19)* have proposed the implementation of a more stringent regulation for medical dispensation of buprenorphine in France than the current general freedom of prescription for all physicians, including practictioners in ambulatory care.

Finally, the high dosage of Subutex tablets is also likely to play a role in the occurrence of accidents, in spite of a theoretical "ceiling effect" (related to the agonist/antagonist duality of buprenorphine pharmacodynamic activity) claimed to reduce this risk *(20)*.

4. CONCLUSION

This chapter has summarized a compendium of 137 fatalities attributed to buprenorphine overdosage recorded in France since the introduction of a high-dosage formulation devoted to the substitution of opiate addicts. This seems to be a specific French problem, since no other deaths have been reported elsewhere.

The risks incurred by the misuse of buprenorphine seem to arise through a combination of two practices: association of other psychotropics, especially benzodiazepines and neuroleptics; and improper use of the tablet form for iv administration or massive oral doses. The demonstration of potentially lethal effects of the buprenorphine-psychotropic(s) association challenges the purported harmlessness of buprenorphine. The total number of buprenorphine-related fatalities in France is probably largely underestimated for these reasons: the drug is difficult to analyze (low concentration, no immunoassay in

France until Spring 2000); only some forensic centers share their data; and in numerous places, in the case of obvious overdose (known drug addict, presence of a syringe or packages of Subutex), no autopsy is requested by the police or a judge.

REFERENCES

1. Marquet P. Pharmacologie de la buprénorphine haut dosage, La Lettre du Pharmacologue 2001;15:40–2.
2. Tracqui A, Petit G, Potard D, Lévy F, Kintz P, Ludes B. Intoxications mortelles par buprénorphine (Subutex) et benzodiazépines: 4 cas. J Med Leg Droit Méd 1997;40:213–23.
3. Tracqui A, Kintz P, Ludes B. Buprenorphine-related deaths among drug addicts in France: a report on 20 fatalities. J Anal Toxicol 1998;22:430–4.
4. Kintz P. Deaths involving buprenorphine: a compendium of French cases, Forensic Sci Int 2001;121:65–9.
5. Auriacombe M, Franques P, Tignol J. Deaths attributable to methadone vs buprenorphine in France, JAMA 2001;285:45.
6. Tracqui A, Kintz P, Mangin P. HPLC/MS determination of buprenorphine and norbuprenorphine in biological fluids and hair samples. J Forensic Sci 1997;42:111–4.
7. Vincent F, Bessard J, Vacheron J, Mallaret M, Bessard G. Determination of buprenorphine and norbuprenorphine in urine and hair by gas chromatography-mass spectrometry. J Anal Toxicol 1999;23:270–9.
8. Hoja H, Marquet P, Verneuil B, Lotfi H, Dupuy JL, Lachatre G. Determination of buprenorphine and norbuprenorphine in whole blood by liquid chromatography-mass spectrometry. J Anal Toxicol 1997;21:160–2.
9. Huestis M. Controlled buprenorphine administration studies. In: Workshop on pharmacology and toxicology of buprenorphine, 52nd annual meeting of the American Academy of Forensic Science, February 21–26, Reno, NV, 2000.
10. Gaulier JM, Marquet P, Lacassie E, Dupuy JL, Lachatre G. Fatal intoxication following self-administration of a massive dose of buprenorphine. J Forensic Sci 2000;45:226–8.
11. Hell RC, Brogden RN, Speight TM, Avery GS. Buprenorphine: a review of its pharmacological properties and therapeutic efficacy. Drugs 1979;17:81–110.
12. Banks CD. Overdosage of buprenorphine: a case report, N Z Med J 1979;89:255–7.
13. Kay B. Buprenorphine, benzodiazepines and respiratory depression. Anaesthesia 1984;39:491–2.
14. Kilicarslan T, Sellers EM. Lack of interaction of buprenorphine with flunitrazepam metabolism. Am J Psychiatry 2000;157:1164–6.
15. Clément R, Fix-Durand MH, Rodat O. Subutex-benzodiazepines, attention danger mortel. Concours Méd 1999;121:915–6.
16. Polettini A, Groppi M. Montagna, The role of alcohol abuse in the etiology of heroin-related deaths. J Anal Toxicol 1999;23:570–6.

17. Downing JW, Goodwin NM, Hicks J. The respiratory depressive effects of intravenous buprenorphine in patients in an intensive care unit. S Afr Med J 1979; 55:1023–7.
18. Pinot JM, Behm J, Robin C, Trapet P. Buprénorphine haut dosage : médicament de substitution ou objet d'addiction? Nervure 2000–2001;13;20–1.
19. Obadia Y, Perrin V, Feroni I, Vlahov D, Moatti JP. Injecting misuse of buprenorphine among French drug users. Addiction 2001;96:267–72.
20. Walsh SL, Preston KL, Stitzer ML, Cone EJ, Bigelow GE. Clinical pharmacology of buprenorphine: ceiling effects at high doses. Clin Pharmacol Ther 1994;55:569–80.

Chapter 9

Pharmacology of Opiates During Pregnancy and in Neonates

Pierre Marquet

1. INTRODUCTION

Opiate addiction in pregnant women and the maintenance treatments that can be proposed to them are two particular cases of regular or iterative chronic dosing of xenobiotics during pregnancy. Moreover, the compounds involved have a predominant neurological action and can influence embryos' development as well as infants' (or even adults') outcome.

Although many mechanisms of action are yet to be discovered and some clinical effects demonstrated, current knowledge allows some evaluation of the potential risks of these compounds resulting from their pharmacokinetic and pharmacodynamic properties, whether in the embryo, the fetus, or the neonate.

2. PERINATAL PHARMACOKINETICS OF OPIATES

2.1. In Utero

2.1.1. Transfer Through Placenta and Distribution in the Fetus

The transfer of drugs and toxicants (*xenobiotics*) from the mother's blood to the fetus through the placenta is either by simple, passive diffusion or through nutrient transfer mechanisms. Small lipophilic molecules, such as opiates (e.g., heroin, morphine, codeine, methadone, buprenorphine), easily cross the thin, lipid-rich membrane constituted by the trophoblastic epithelium and the vascular endothelium of the placenta villi, inasmuch as the exchange surface area is large and blood flows are high on both sides *(1)*. Such compounds are there-

From *Forensic Science and Medicine: Buprenorphine Therapy of Opiate Addiction*
Edited by: P. Kintz and P. Marquet © Humana Press Inc., Totowa, NJ

fore brought through the umbilical vein, partly toward the systemic circulation via the ductus venosus and partly to the fetus's liver, where they are submitted to a hepatic first-pass effect before entering the systemic circulation. Nevertheless, this hepatic metabolism is generally weaker than in infants or adults, because the enzymes involved (cytochromes P450 and UDP-glucuronyl-transferases) are only progressively expressed and activated during gestation. The elimination of these compounds in urine, which, in adults, essentially concerns metabolites, is also less efficient in the fetus, because of immature renal function (the renal blood flow represents 3% of systemic flow rate vs 25% in adults, and the tubular excretion of acids is inefficient) and because the fraction eliminated in the amniotic fluid is partly reabsorbed by fetal swallowing. There is, therefore, a risk of accumulation of these drugs, but this risk is theoretically limited by the passive equilibrium of their nonionized, free fraction between the fetal and the maternal blood. However, the total body content is dependent on protein binding and pH-dependent ionization of these drugs, and these are obviously different in the fetus and the mother, lower blood concentrations of proteins and lipoproteins not favoring, and lower blood pH favoring accumulation of basic drugs in the neonate *(2)*.

2.1.2. Transfer Through Blood-Brain Barrier

In adults, the blood-brain barrier is permeable to small, lipid-soluble molecules, which explains the rapid and intense psychotropic effects of opiates. Because this barrier is much more permeable in the fetus and the neonate, the distribution of these compounds to the brain is even easier.

2.2. Postnatal

In the neonate, the absorption of opiates is through breast feeding or, as far as therapeutic administration of morphine or paregoric is concerned, generally by the digestive route. Because some enzymatic systems are immature in the neonate, the first-pass effect of opiates, resulting in partial inactivation, is weaker than in adults and bioavailability is higher. On the other hand, as in the fetus, the transfer of opiates through the blood-brain barrier is easier than in adults.

3. Perinatal Pharmacodynamics of Opiates

3.1. Opioid Receptors and Development of Embryos

In pigs, during *in utero* development, the δ opioid receptors modulate the waking and sleeping behaviors, and the μ opioid receptors modulate respiration, a specificity that attenuates during development *(3)*. In rats, both systems play a part in the electroencephalographic activity *(4)*, while, during the prenatal phase, the μ and κ systems influence and modulate the development of suckling attitudes and mother-fetus interactions *(5)*. Blocking of the opioid receptors by naltrexone during the entire gestation period induces an increase in birth weight, accelerates the postnatal apparition of motor behavior and reflexes, while inhibiting other behaviors: the opioid system would thus influence somatic, physical, and behavioral development *(6)*; it is regarded as a mediator of growth and functions of brain tissue, but it also acts on cellular proliferation in the retina *(7)*, uterus *(8)*, or other organs *(9)*. β-Endorphin also influences human chorionic gonadotropin (hCG) secretion by the early stage placenta *(10)*, which has been confirmed in vitro by incubation of first-trimester and third-trimester trophoblasts with morphine: hCG secretion increased in the former but not in the latter *(11)*.

3.2. Perinatal Effects of Exogenous Opiates

3.2.1. On Development

Opiates decrease the active placental transfer of amino acids, owing to their effects on opioid (stimulation of κ receptors) and above all cholinergic systems (inhibition of acetylcholine release) that regulate this transport. This could partly explain the growth retardation noticed with these drugs *(12)*.

The administration of morphine to female rats during the entire pregnancy reduced the number of neurons in the primary somatosensory cortex *(13)* and that of cholinergic neurons in the frontal cortex, brain stem, and medulla in the neonate *(14)*. On the other hand, the perinatal administration of a specific agonist of κ receptors in rats altered the development of dopamine receptors and of motor behaviors mediated by dopamine *(15)*.

Although high-dose methadone is teratogenic in certain animal species, mainly inducing encephalopathies and central nervous system abnormalities *(16,17)*, it does not seem to be associated with inborn abnormalities in humans, in whom it has been used over the past three decades, particularly in the United States. Buprenorphine was not found to be teratogenic in the animal species in which it was tested, but at very high doses in the rats it increases perinatal death rate *(18)*. The common effects of methadone and buprenorphine in newborns are low birthweight (though generally not so much as under heroin) and withdrawal syndromes.

Finally, an epidemiological study demonstrated that the risk of becoming a drug addict during adult life was significantly increased in individuals exposed to opiates, barbiturates, or nitrous oxide at birth, during labor *(19)*.

3.2.2. On Opioid System

In animal experiments, prenatal exposure to low doses of psychotropic drugs (methadone, diazepam) induced an abnormal behavioral development *(20)*. At the physiopathological level, it was demonstrated that administration of buprenorphine (an agonist-antagonist of opioid receptors) in pregnant rats induced a decrease in the density of brain µ receptors density in themselves and in their offspring. In newborns, this abnormality was found on the first day of life but not on the seventh *(21)*. On the contrary, brain levels of enkephalins were not affected by buprenorphine, whereas they were significantly decreased in groups administered methadone *(22)*. Finally, the newborn rat is more sensitive than the adult to the analgesic effect of opiates, but the relative potency of the different compounds of this class is unchanged *(23)*.

4. MAINTENANCE TREATMENTS DURING PREGNANCY

The few published studies on drug withdrawal in pregnant women showed a high relapse rate. Only a small proportion of highly motivated expectant mothers seem to be capable of total abstinence. The others relapse into drug abuse with its cycles of intoxication and withdrawal periods accompanied by large variations in opiate blood concentrations, which may have a severe impact on fetal development *(24)*. Therefore, a maintenance treatment by an opiate seems preferable, despite the potential risks of these compounds. Only methadone seems to be licensed for this purpose worldwide, even in those countries, such as France, where buprenorphine has been routinely used as a maintenance drug for some years. However, since there are about 10 times more patients on buprenorphine than on methadone maintenance in the particular case of France (64,300 and 7150 in 1998, respectively), a nonnegligible number of pregnancies occurred in buprenorphine-maintained women. Moreover, owing to the relative innocuity of the drug in most drug addicts and to the reassuring first case reports, buprenorphine maintenance was prescribed in a nonnegligible number of pregnant drug addicts. We reported the first toxicologically documented case of buprenorphine withdrawal syndrome in a newborn *(25)* and, more recently, the results of clinical and toxicological investigations in 6 *(26)* and 14 newborns *(27)* exposed to high-dose buprenorphine *in utero*. Since then, several other such cases have been registered by the French pharmacovigilance network, but generally without toxicological confirmation.

REFERENCES

1. Morgan DJ. Drug disposition in mothers and fœtus. Clin Exp Pharmacol Physiol 1997;24:869–73.
2. Garland M. Pharmacology of drug transfer across the placenta. Obstet Gynecol Clin North Am 1998;25:21–42.
3. Moss IR, Scott SC, Inman JD. Mu- vs. delta-opioid influence on respiratory and sleep behavior during development. Am J Physiol 1993;264:R754–60.
4. Cheng PY, Wu D, Soong Y, McCabe S, Deneca JA, Szeto HH. Role of mu 1- and delta-opioid receptors in modulation of fetal EEG and respiratory activity. Am J Physiol 1993;265:R433–:8.
5. Smotherman WP, Simonik DK, Andersen SL, Robinson SR. Mu and kappa opioid systems modulate responses to cutaneous stimulation in the fetal rat. Physiol Behav 1993;53:751–6.
6. Mac Laughlin PJ, Tobias SW, Lang CM, Zagon IS. Opioid receptor blockade during prenatal life modifies postnatal behavioral development. Pharmacol Biochem Behav 1997;58:1075–82.
7. Isayama T, McLaughlin PJ, Zagon IS. Endogenous opioids regulate cell proliferation in the retina of developing rat. Brain Res 1991;544:79–85.
8. Vertes Z, Kornyei JL, Kovacs S, Vertes M. Opioids regulate cell proliferation in the developing rat uterus: effects during the period of sexual maturation. J Steroid Biochem Mol Biol 1996;59:173–8.
9. Zagon IS, Wu Y, McLaughlin PJ. Opioid growth factor and organ development in rat and human embryos. Brain Res 1999;839:313–22.
10. Barnea ER, Ashkenazy R, Tal Y, Kol S, Sarne Y. Effect of beta-endorphin on human chorionic gonadotrophin secretion by placental explants. Hum Reprod 1991; 6:1327–31.
11. Cemerikic B, Genbacev O, Sulovic V, Beaconsfield R. Effect of morphine on hCG release by first trimester human trophoblast in vitro. Life Sci 1988;42:1773–9.
12. Sastry BV. Placental toxicology: tobacco smoke, abused drugs, multiple chemical interactions, and placental function. Reprod Fertil Dev 1991;3:355–72.
13. Seatriz JV, Hammer RPJr. Effects of opiates on neuronal development in the rat cerebral cortex. Brain Res Bull 1993;30:523–7.
14. Miller JH, Azmitia EC. Growth inhibitory effects of a mu opioid on cultured cholinergic neurons from fetal rat ventral forebrain, brainstem, and spinal cord. Brain Res Dev Brain Res 1999;114:69–77.
15. Shieh GJ, Walters DE. Altered neurochemical and behavioral development of 10-day-old rats perinatally exposed to the kappa opioid agonist U-50,488H. Neurosci Lett 1994;176:37–40.
16. Geber WF, Schramm LC. Congenital malformations of the central nervous system produced by narcotic analgesics in the hamster. Am J Obstet Gynecol 1975; 123:705–13.
17. Jurand A. Teratogenic activity of methadone hydrochloride in mouse and chicken embryos. J Embryol Exp Morph 1973;30:449–58.

18. Evans RG, Olley JE, Rice GE, Abrahams JM. Effects of subacute opioid administration during late pregnancy in the rat on the initiation, duration and outcome of parturition and maternal levels of oxytocin and arginine vasopressin. Clin Exp Pharmacol Physiol 1989;16:169–78.
19. Jacobson B, Nyberg K, Gronbladh L, Eklund G, Bydeman M, Rydberg U. Opiate addiction in adult offspring through possible imprinting after obstetric treatment. BMJ 1990;301:1067–70.
20. Perry BD, Pesavento DJ, Kussie PH, U'Pichard DC, Schnoll SH. Prenatal exposure to drugs of abuse in humans: effects on placental neurotransmitter receptors. Neurobehav Toxicol Teratol 1984;6:295–301.
21. Belcheva MM, Dawn S, Barg J, McHale RJ, Ho MT, Ignatova E, Coscia CJ. Transient down-regulation of neonatal rat brain μ-opioid receptors upon in utero exposure to buprenorphine. Dev Brain Res 1994;80:158–62.
22. Tiong GKL, Olley JE. Effects of exposure in utero to methadone and buprenorphine on enkephalin levels in the developing rat brain. Neurosci Lett 1988;93:101–6.
23. McLaughlin CR, Dewey WL. A comparison of the antinociceptive effects of opioid antagonists in neonatal and adult rats in phasic and tonic nociceptive tests. Pharmacol Biochem Behav 1994;49:1017–23.
24. Jarvis MAE, Schnoll SH. Methadone treatment during pregnancy. J Psychoact Drugs 1994;26:155–61.
25. Marquet P, Chevrel J, Lavignasse P, Merle L, Lachâtre G. Buprenorphine withdrawal syndrome in a newborn. Clin Pharmacol Ther 1997;62:569–71.
26. Marquet P, Lavignasse P, Chevrel J, Merle L, Lachâtre G. Exposition au SUBUTEX® in utero et syndrome de manque du nouveau-né. Toxicorama 1999;11:17–24.
27. Marquet P. High-dose buprenorphine (HD-BU) use in pregnant women and consequences for their newborn. In: Proceedings of the 52nd annual meeting of the American Academy of Forensic Sciences, Reno, NV, February 21–26, 2000.

Chapter 10

Case Study of Neonates Born to Mothers Undergoing Buprenorphine Maintenance Treatment

Pierre Marquet, Pierre Lavignasse, Jean-Michel Gaulier, and Gérard Lachâtre

1. INTRODUCTION

In 2000 in France there were over 60,000 ex-drug addicts undergoing high-dose buprenorphine maintenance, to whom must be added those who illicitly use this drug after buying it in the street. It is thus probable that a nonnegligible number of expectant mothers can be found among these buprenorphine users. The literature is poor on the effects of this drug in the fetus *(1,2)*, as well as the effects of the brutal cessation of exposure at birth. The results of animal studies, reported in the introductive chapter (Chapter 9), showed the absence of teratogenic and embryotoxic effects in the animal species in which it was tested.

Based on the findings of previous case reports *(3–6)*, we and others were able to confirm the transfer of buprenorphine through the placenta in humans, which was most likely at the theoretical and clinical levels. Additionally, these cases allowed us to attribute unambiguously some of the withdrawal syndromes diagnosed in neonates to high-dose buprenorphine alone, since we were able to demonstrate that they were exposed to no other opiate nor to benzodiazepines during the last weeks of pregnancy.

We report here the results of a case-control study that we undertook using a compendium of 23 cases of neonates born to mothers undergoing

From *Forensic Science and Medicine: Buprenorphine Therapy of Opiate Addiction*
Edited by: P. Kintz and P. Marquet © Humana Press Inc., Totowa, NJ

buprenorphine maintenance during pregnancy. This is a first step (and probably the last, because it is the only ethical one) in the evaluation of the respective responsibilities of buprenorphine maintenance and opiates sometimes abused by the mothers on the incidence and severity of withdrawal syndrome in the neonates.

2. CLINICAL FINDINGS

2.1. Neonates Included

In this study were included all the neonates born to mothers undergoing high-dose buprenorphine maintenance treatment for at least the last 4 mo of pregnancy and from whom urine or meconium samples were collected in the first 24 h of life (however, always before withdrawal signs were noticed) for toxicological investigation. They were from different regions of France but mainly from the southwest (Côte Basque Hospital, Bayonne), where the addiction maintenance center is run by a nongovernment association, Médecin du Monde. Contacts between the Department of Pharmacology and Toxicology and the physicians were generally established before parturition, with the aim of standardizing data and sample collection as well as the clinical monitoring of the neonate (by means of the Finnegan score). Two questionnaires were sent to the physicians in charge of the mother and the neonate, the first one concerning the mother's drug addiction and maintenance treatment and the second the newborn's circumstances of birth, health, and outcome (mainly regarding withdrawal signs).

The present compendium comprises 23 mothers and their 23 infants. On the day of parturition, the mothers' drug addiction history was 1–20 yr long and the mothers had been under high-dose buprenorphine treatment for the previous 5 mo to 4 yr. They were administered 1–16 mg/d of buprenorphine (average daily dose at the end of pregnancy was 5.6 mg), with progressive tapering during pregnancy in two of them (Table 1). In one case (case B), buprenorphine maintenance had been interrupted for the final 6 wk before parturition but probably not the abuse of buprenorphine (though not admitted by the patient), as suggested by the presence of buprenorphine and norbuprenorphine in all the samples collected in the neonate. Consequently, this case was included in this study.

2.2. Questionnaire and Toxicological Survey of Mothers

The questionnaires applied to the mothers revealed the following data: tobacco smoking ($\geq$10 cigarettes/d) in 16 of 17 patients who answered; abuse

Table 1
Summary of Questionnaires

Case no.	Daily dose of buprenorphine	Survey of drug abuse during pregnancy — Acknowledged abuse	Survey of drug abuse during pregnancy — Urine screening	Withdrawal syndrome — Finnegan score and time of occurrence	Withdrawal syndrome — Treatment	Screening of drugs after childbirth — Mothers' urine	Screening of drugs after childbirth — Newborns' urine	Screening of drugs after childbirth — Newborns' meconium
A	4 mg	—	Always negative	FS > 8 from h 48 to h70	None	Absence	Absence	Absence
B	6 mg, terminated 6 wk before childbirth	—	None	FS < 8	None	—	Absence	—
C	4 mg	—	Always negative	FS = 13 on d4	—	—	Absence	Absence
D	8 mg	Cocaine occasionally at mo 6 and 7. Oral morphine for 1 wk at mo 8	None	FS = 16 at h22	Oral morphine from h22 to d6 + diazepam from d3 to d10	BZE, EME (hair; codeine, morphine)	(hair; codeine, morphine)	—
E	6 mg	Heroin intravenously 3–4 times per mo	Cocaine once	FS >20 on d1	—	Absence	Absence	Morphine Codeine
F	Tapered down from 8 to 2 mg	—	None	<8	None	Absence	Absence	Absence
G	1.2 mg	Buprenorphine intravenously sporadically	Always negative	<8	None	—	Absence	Absence
H	16 mg	Buprenorphine intravenously, regularly	Always negative	FS = 7 at h44 FS = 13 at h55 FS = 12 at h58 FS = 13 at h59 FS = 0 at d16	Oral morphine from d4 to d16	Cannabinoids	Cannabinoids	—

Table 1 (continued)
Summary of Questionnaires

Case no.	Daily dose of buprenorphine	Survey of drug abuse during pregnancy — Acknowledged abuse	Survey of drug abuse during pregnancy — Urine screening	Withdrawal syndrome — Finnegan score and time of occurrence	Withdrawal syndrome — Treatment	Screening of drugs after childbirth — Mothers' urine^a	Screening of drugs after childbirth — Newborns' urine	Screening of drugs after childbirth — Newborns' meconium
I	10 mg	Buprenorphine intravenously sporadically	—	FS = 13 on d5	Oral morphine for 20 d, then chlorpromazine for 16 d	Benzodiazepines	Benzodiazepines	Absence
J	2 mg	—	—	FS >8 from d2 to d3	—	Cannabinoids	Cannabinoids	Cannabinoids
K	16 mg	Buprenorphine intravenously, intermittently	None	FS = 10 on d3	Oral morphine for 1 mo	Benzodiazepines	—	Absence
L	1 mg	Buprenorphine intravenously, intermittently, on mo 2 and 4	—	FS ≥10 on d3 (h86)	Oral morphine: 0.6 mL four times daily for >13 d	Cannabinoids	—	Cannabinoids
M	8 mg	Cannabis smoking	None	<8	None	Cannabinoids Opiates (6-MAM; morphine)	Cannabinoids Opiates (morphine)	Cannabinoids No opiates (confirmed by GC-MS)
N	2 mg	None	None	<8	None	Methadone Cannabinoids	Absence	Opiates (morphine) Cannabinoids
O	8 mg	Buprenorphine intravenously twice daily	None	FS = 12 on d1 FS = 21 on d2 FS = 11 on d4	Oral morphine 0.15 mg/kg every 6 h for 21 d, then progressive tapering	—	Opiates (morphine) Cannabinoids	Cannabinoids

P	Tapered down from 6 to 4 mg at mo 7	Cannabis smoking	Cannabinoids once	<8	None	Cannabinoids	—	Cannabinoids
Q	2 mg	Heroin intravenously once a wk Cannabis smoking every day Alcohol during first 6 mo	Always negative	FS = 17 on d4	Oral morphine on d4 (unknown duration)	Absence	Absence	Opiates (morphine) Cannabinoids
R	—	—	None	—	—	Opiates (morphine) Cannabinoids	Cannabinoids	—
S	2 mg	None	None	<8	None	—	Absence	Cannabinoids
T	—	—	None	—	—	—	Absence	Absence
U	10 mg	Buprenorphine intravenously 3 times daily	Cocaine Cannabinoids	FS = 13 on d1 FS = 17 on d2	None	Cocaine, BZE, EME Cannabinoids	Cocaine, BZE, EME Cannabinoids	Cocaine, BZE, EME Cannabinoids
V	2 mg 3 times a day	None	None	FS = 12 only once on d1	None	Absence	Absence	Absence
W	4 mg	Cannabis once a wk	Cannabinoids 3 times Cocaine and opiates once	FS =11 and 14 on d2	None	Cannabinoids Ethanol (0.6 g/L)	Cannabinoids	Cannabinoids

h, hour(s); d, day(s)
— = missing data.
BZE, benzoylecgonine and EME, ecgonine methyl ester, cocaine metabolites; 6-MAM, monoacetyl-6-morphine, primary heroine metabolite.

of opiates, alcohol, or illicit drugs in 13 of 16 patients who answered (buprenorphine intravenously in 7 cases, cannabis in 4, heroin in 2, morphine in 1, cocaine in 1, alcohol in 1), therapeutic drug use, mostly under prescriptions, by 5 of 15 patients (benzodiazepines three times; antidepressants twice; meprobamate, a carbamate tranquilizer, once). Drug screening was performed on the urine of 9 expectant mothers and positive results were found in 4 (3 times for cannabis, 3 for cocaine, once for opiates, and none for amphetamines) (Table 1).

2.3. Neonates' Outcomes

No abnormality was found in any neonate. Birth weight was generally low, ranging from 1.70 to 3.89 kg (mean = 2.77 kg). The Apgar vitality score was maximal at min 5 in 20 of 21 neonates in whom this value could be obtained, and suboptimal in one (Apgar = 8).

The apparition of a withdrawal syndrome was monitored using the Finnegan score, which is based on different, mainly neurological, digestive, and sympathetic clinical signs *(7)*. This score ranges between 0 and 40 and theoretically indicates withdrawal when it is higher than 8 on three successive occasions, measured at 20-min intervals. Of 21 evaluable cases (Table 1): no withdrawal syndrome was noted in 8 cases (38%) (group I); a mild and early withdrawal syndrome was found in 3 neonates (14%) for whom nursing was sufficient, so that no pharmacological treatment had to be administered (group II); and moderate to severe withdrawal was found in 10 cases (47%) (group III), during the first 24 h for 3 of them and after 44 h in the others (mean: 33.1 h). The treatment of withdrawal is unknown in three neonates of group III, while morphine hydrochloride was administered orally in the seven others, followed by chlorpromazine in one case and diazepam in another. The length of this treatment in six cases in which it is known with precision ranged from 1 to 36 d (mean: 16.5 d).

3. TOXICOLOGICAL INVESTIGATIONS

3.1. Material and Methods

Buprenorphine and norbuprenorphine were screened for and determined in mothers', neonates', and umbilical cord serum, as well as in newborns' urine and meconium by liquid chromatography-mass spectrometry (LC-MS), following previously published techniques *(8,9)*.

Opiates, amphetamines, cocaine metabolites, cannabinoids, and benzodiazepines were screened for in mothers' and neonates' urine as well as in meconium by fluorescence polarization immunoassays using an AxSYM automaton. The positive results were confirmed by gas chromatography-ms (GC-

MS) following the methods recommended by the French Society of Analytical Toxicology *(10–12)*, except for benzodiazepines, which were determined by high performance liquid chromatography coupled to diode-array ultraviolet detection. Opiates in hair were directly determined by GC-MS following another consensus method *(13)*.

3.2. Results

Buprenorphine and norbuprenorphine concentrations in mothers' serum sampled after childbirth showed a large interindividual variability (Table 2), probably owing to a highly variable time lag between the last dose of buprenorphine and sampling. In the four cases in which cord blood was sampled, it is noteworthy that buprenorphine and norbuprenorphine concentrations were generally lower than those measured in the respective mothers' blood (buprenorphine = 1.36 vs 5.42 ng/mL; norbuprenorphine = 3.46 vs 13.95 ng/mL, on average). Blood samples were collected from nine infants, from 1 h to 3 d after birth. On average, serum concentrations were of the same order as cord and lower than mothers' serum concentrations (buprenorphine = 2.03 ng/mL; norbuprenorphine = 4.84 ng/mL). In case B, in which the maintenance treatment was terminated 6 wk before childbirth, blood levels of buprenorphine and norbuprenorphine were, respectively, 3.3 and 3.0 ng/mL in the neonate (i.e., close to the average values), suggesting high-dose buprenorphine abuse by the mother. Unfortunately, no blood or urine samples were collected from the latter.

Buprenorphine and norbuprenorphine concentrations in newborns' blood only tended to be correlated with the dose, probably owing to the limited number of values ($n = 9$), whereas norbuprenorphine concentrations in maternal serum were significantly correlated with the administered dose ($r = 0.75; p = 0.0042; n = 12$). On the other hand, no correlation could be found between buprenorphine and norbuprenorphine concentrations in maternal blood and those in the neonatal or cord blood, possibly also owing to a lack of statistical power.

Buprenorphine and norbuprenorphine concentrations in mothers' and newborns' urine as well as in meconium samples showed a high interindividual variability (Table 2) that cannot be explained by the dose administered (with which these concentrations are not correlated), except for norbuprenorphine in maternal urine. As in serum, urine levels were lower in the neonates than in the mothers. The meconium levels were of intermediate value. Moreover, the mean metabolic ratio (norbuprenorphine:buprenorphine) was higher in mothers' than in newborns' urine (3.0 and 1.7 respectively), but similar in serum (maternal blood: 2.6; cord blood: 2.5; neonatal blood: 2.4); this ratio was 1.4 in meconium.

Illicit drug screening and confirmation were performed on the 17 maternal urine samples available (Table 1), showing negative results in five cases

Table 2
Buprenorphine and Norbuprenorphine Concentrations in Serum, Urine, and Meconium

	Withdrawal +			Withdrawal −			Global mean	Global CV (%)	Correlation with dose (r)	Mann-Whitney U test between two subgroups
	n	Mean	CV (%)	n	Mean	CV (%)				
Buprenorphine dose at end of pregnancy (mg/d)	13	7.25	70.36	6	3.20	79.06	**5.82**	75.63	—	0.153 (NS)
Maternal serum										
buprenorphine (ng/mL)	8	6.50	135.59	4	3.29	134.32	**5.42**	139.53	0.27 (NS)	0.396 (NS)
norbuprenorphine (ng/mL)	8	18.76	119.33	4	4.32	117.48	**13.95**	139.14	**0.76** (**p < 0.005**)	0.089 (NS)
Cord serum										
buprenorphine (ng/mL)	3	1.68	107.60	1	0.40	—	**1.36**	118.32	−0.11 (NS)	0.655 (NS)
norbuprenorphine (ng/mL)	3	4.01	114.20	1	1.80	—	**3.46**	112.77	−0.12 (NS)	0.655 (NS)
Neonatal serum										
buprenorphine (ng/mL)	6	1.91	90.12	3	2.27	86.71	**2.03**	83.20	0.56 (NS)	0.796 (NS)
norbuprenorphine (ng/mL)	6	5.07	110.10	3	4.40	119.14	**4.84**	106.12	0.56 (NS)	0.897 (NS)
Maternal urine										
buprenorphine (ng/mL)	5	532.55	102.55	5	191.20	96.64	**361.87**	117.27	0.22 (NS)	0.465 (NS)
norbuprenorphine (ng/mL)	5	1646.06	180.67	5	521.50	134.22	**1083.78**	195.73	0.58 (p = 0.06; NS)	0.584 (NS)
Neonatal urine										
buprenorphine (ng/mL)	6	56.67	135.60	5	17.46	80.71	**36.68**	154.06	0.22 (NS)	0.465 (NS)
norbuprenorphine (ng/mL)	6	65.49	119.05	5	62.65	101.67	**62.79**	104.00	0.27 (NS)	0.855 (NS)
Meconium										
buprenorphine (ng/g)	9	202.36	140.15	6	27.41	159.41	**121.91**	180.89	0.33 (NS)	0.059 (NS)
norbuprenorphine (ng/g)	9	261.20	88.50	6	72.25	137.70	**176.22**	111.56	0.21 (NS)	0.126 (NS)

and revealing the presence of opiates in two (heroine intake once and methadone abuse once), cocaine metabolites in two, cannabinoids in nine, benzodiazepines in two and ethanol in one.

The screening procedures in newborns' urine, meconium, and/or hair revealed negative results in eight cases, of which there was one discrepant result between mother and newborn (case K): benzodiazepines were found in the mother's urine sample, collected after a cesarian section, while no trace of benzodiazepines could be detected in the neonate's urine and meconium, thus suggesting administration of a benzodiazepine during surgery, immediately before birth. Opiates could be found in six newborns' samples, including morphine alone in four cases and morphine and codeine in two. Cocaine metabolites were found in urine and meconium of a single newborn and cannabinoids were present in 12 cases, more often in meconium (10 times) than in urine (6 times). Finally, benzodiazepines were found only once, in a urine sample.

4. DISCUSSION

Despite the still small number of clinical cases in which convenient samples could be obtained, it seems that a nonnegligible number of pregnant women on maintenance treatment with high-dose buprenorphine keep abusing illicit or therapeutic psychotropic drugs, as is the case for those treated with methadone *(14)*. This should lead to more systematic and more frequent urine screening for these compounds during pregnancy. When this screening was performed in the present cases, it allowed unacknowledged abuse to be detected, particularly cocaine (three cases)—though its use is still infrequent in France—and opiates (one case). Inversely, whether before or after childbirth, these urine assays were negative for opiates in two cases in which the mothers had admitted to continuing injecting heroin (cases E and Q) and in which opiates were found in newborns' hair or meconium samples. This finding points to the relative shortness of the detection window for these drugs in urine and to the interest of meconium or hair for drug screening. However, if in four cases psychotropic drugs were detected in meconium but not in neonatal urine, the reverse situation was found five times. Both types of samples thus seem complementary for evaluating *in utero* exposure to psychotropic drugs.

Mothers whose babies presented a withdrawal syndrome ($n = 13$) received a mean buprenorphine dose of 7.25 mg/J, vs 3.60 mg/d in the others ($n = 8$), but this difference is not statistically significant ($p = 0.17$), probably due to small numbers. Mean serum concentrations of buprenorphine and norbuprenorphine tended to be higher in the first group than in the second, while no tendency was obvious as far as cord and newborns' serum were concerned.

In urine and meconium samples of the neonates who presented a withdrawal syndrome and in the urine samples of their mothers, mean levels of buprenorphine and norbuprenorphine tended to be higher than in the samples of the other neonates and mothers (Table 2). On the other hand, the fact that the metabolic ratio (norbuprenorphine:buprenorphine) was lower in neonatal urine or meconium than in maternal urine but equivalent in serum samples suggests incomplete renal elimination rather than immature metabolism. Nevertheless, a part of norbuprenorphine detected in neonatal serum could come from maternal blood through the placenta, so metabolic immaturity could be superimposed on limited elimination.

Among the six newborns who were exposed *in utero* to opiates other than buprenorphine, two showed no withdrawal signs, three presented a moderate to severe withdrawal syndrome, and in the last case clinical information was too limited. Withdrawal signs were precocious (<24 h) in two cases and late (d 4) in the third case. In the absence of drug abuse (16 cases), high-dose buprenorphine maintenance treatment induced a withdrawal syndrome in 10 infants (63%), occurring generally late (beyond the h 44 in 8 cases) and of variable intensity, from mild to severe.

5. Conclusion

This case study gives clues to the nature and frequency of abuse of psychoactive drugs by the mothers on high-dose buprenorphine maintenance treatment, on the health status of the newborns at birth, and on the frequency and delay of withdrawal attributable to high-dose buprenorphine or to high-dose buprenorphine plus other drugs. Despite persistent drug abuse in several cases, this study allows the use of high-dose buprenorphine to be envisaged as a maintenance treatment for pregnant women addicted to heroin, as an alternative to methadone, which frequently induces withdrawal syndrome of mild to high severity in the newborn *(14)*. Buprenorphine induced no teratogenic nor embryotoxic effects. The overall rate of withdrawal syndrome was 62%, whether buprenorphine was associated with other opiates or not. Withdrawal from buprenorphine alone seemed to occur later than buprenorphine with other opiates, with no marked difference in intensity. This is consistent with the respective pharmacokinetic and pharmacodynamic properties of buprenorphine and of morphine and codeine. This study points out the usefulness of toxicological investigations to detect drug abuse in expectant mothers, which may be responsible for or favor withdrawal in the neonate. However, further studies are needed to evaluate whether the association of buprenorphine and other opiates leads to more frequent withdrawal than buprenorphine alone.

ACKNOWLEDGMENTS

We particularly thank the pediatricians, gynecologists, and biologists from the hospitals of Bayonne, Dax, Le Mans, Limoges, Nancy, Poitiers, and Rouen for their collaboration.

REFERENCES

1. Boobis AR, Burley D, Margerison Davies D, Davies DS, Harrison PI, Orme ME, Park BK, Goldberg LI. Buprenorphine. In: Therapeutic drugs, vol. 1, Dollery C, ed., Kent, UK, Churchill Livingstone, 1991.
2. Committee on Drugs of the American Academy of Pediatrics. Neonatal drug withdrawal. Pediatrics 1998;101:1079–88.
3. Marquet P, Chevrel J, Lavignasse P, Merle L, Lachâtre G. Buprenorphine withdrawal syndrome in a newborn. Clin Pharmacol Ther 1997;62:569–71.
4. Jernite M, Viville B, Escande B, Brettes JP, Messer J. Grossesse et buprénorphine. À propos de 24 cas. Arch Pediatr 1999;6:1179–89.
5. Marquet P, Lavignasse P, Chevrel J, Merle L, Lachâtre G. Exposition au Subutex in utero et syndrome de manque du nouveau-né. Toxicorama 1999;11:17–24.
6. Marquet P. High-dose buprenorphine use in pregnant women and consequences for their newborn. In: Proceedings of the 52nd Annual Meeting of the American Academy of Forensic Sciences, Reno, NV, February 21–24, 2000.
7. Finnegan LP, Weiner SM. Drug withdrawal in the neonate. In: Neonatal intensive care. Merenstein GB, Gardner SL, eds., New York: Mosby Year Book, 1993.
8. Hoja H, Marquet P, Verneuil B, Lotfi H, Dupuy J-L, Dreyfuss M-F, Lachâtre G. Dosage de buprénorphine et de norbuprénorphine dans l'urine et le sérum par chromatographie liquide couplée à la spectrométrie de masse avec ionisation de type électrospray. Analusis 1996;24:104–7.
9. Hoja H, Marquet P, Verneuil B, Lotfi H, Dupuy J-L, Lachâtre G. Determination of buprenorphine and norbuprenorphine in whole blood samples by liquid chromatography mass spectrometry. J Anal Toxicol 1997;21:160–5.
10. Kintz P, Cirimele V, Pépin G, Marquet P, Deveaux M, Mura P. Identification et dosage des cannabinoides dans le sang total. Toxicorama 1996;8(2):8–10.
11. Gaillard Y, Pépin G, Marquet P, Kintz P, Deveaux M, Mura P. Identification et dosage de benzoylecgonine, cocaïne, méthylecgonine-ester, codéine, morphine et 6-acétylmorphine dans le sang total. Toxicorama 1996;8:17–22.
12. Marquet P, Lachâtre G, Kintz P, Pépin G, Deveaux M, Mura P. Identification et dosage des principales drogues amphétaminiques dans le sang total par chromatographie en phase gazeuse couplée à la spectrométrie de masse (CPG-SM). Toxicorama 1996;8(2):23–8.
13. Cirimele V, Kintz P, Tracqui A, Mangin P. Comparaison des techniques d'extraction de la cocaïne et des opiacés dans les cheveux. Toxicorama 1994;6(1):1–10.
14. Jarvis M-A-E, Schnoll S-H. Methadone treatment during pregnancy. J Psychoactive Drugs 1994;26:155–6.

Chapter 11

Buprenorphine and Pregnancy

A Comparative, Multicenter Clinical Study of High-Dose Buprenorphine vs Methadone Maintenance

Claude Lejeune, Sandrine Aubisson, Laurence Simmat-Durand, Fabrice Cneude, and Martine Piquet

1. INTRODUCTION

The perinatal prognosis for drug-addicted pregnant women and their children is clearly improved by a specialized treatment of their addiction, of which an essential element is the prescription of a substitute along with the necessary medico- and psychosocial support, and by early supervision of the pregnancy *(1–3)*. Even though the prescription of high doses of buprenorphine is, in principle, not approved in France during pregnancy, the small number of openings available in methadone centers and more liberal prescription rules for high-dose buprenorphine mean, in practice, that numerous pregnant, drug-addicted women are having their treatment substituted with high-dose buprenorphine.

There are far fewer studies concerning the use of high-dose buprenorphine when compared to methadone, but the prognosis for pregnancy seems to have improved *(4–7)*. The neonatal withdrawal syndrome in children with mothers under methadone or high-dose buprenorphine appears to be relatively severe *(4,8)* and probably more intense under methadone than heroin. In the absence of data on the outcome of pregnancies under methadone or high-dose buprenorphine, there is, for the moment, no consensus on the substitution treatment to be administered during pregnancy. The object of this study was to

From *Forensic Science and Medicine: Buprenorphine Therapy of Opiate Addiction*
Edited by: P. Kintz and P. Marquet © Humana Press Inc., Totowa, NJ

compare perinatal morbidity and neonatal withdrawal syndrome in children of mothers taking methadone or high-dose buprenorphine during pregnancy.

2. MATERIAL AND METHODS

This prospective study was carried out by the Groupe d'Etudes Grossesse et Addictions (GEGA) from the January 10, 1998 to the March 9, 1999. Included were all children born during this period in the 34 French centers participating (list annexed) whose mothers received a substitution treatment during pregnancy, whether it started before or during pregnancy; the treatment had to be prescribed within a protocol, i.e., within the confines of a close relationship with a specialized center or general practitioner and followed right up until birth. The sociodemographic data concerning the family, the progress of the pregnancy, their behavior as addicts (on a declarative basis), and the outcome for the newborn were collected prospectively. The intensity of the neonatal withdrawal syndrome was evaluated by its Lipsitz score *(9)* as recommended by the American Academy of Paediatrics *(10)*. The choice of medical treatment of the syndrome was left to the teams concerned.

The care of pregnant woman addicts has been markedly humanized over the past few years on the part of the teams participating in this study. The changes in practices concern the following points.

1. The care of these pregnancies as ones at risk of perinatal complications with no reference to the illegal use of drugs. Close and early prenatal care leads to prevention of most of the usual perinatal complications, prematurity in particular. A retrospective study carried out from 1988 to 1993 in the north of les Hauts de Seine (the suburban low-socioeconomic population of a Paris district) showed, in the absence of structured care, catastrophic results on the social level, with, according to the latest information, only one-third of children being brought up by their mother *(11)*. Analysis of this cohort and relevant literature *(2,11,12)* shows that the outcome for these children depends essentially on the quality of their environment and pathologies indirectly linked to the consumption of heroin (prematurity, human immunodeficiency virus [HIV] infection, and the consequences of taking alcohol or cocaine for the fetus). The incidence of perinatal complications (such as prematurity, low birth weight, acute fetal distress, transmission of HIV) can be diminished if these pregnancies are properly supervised and if the addict is cared for by specialists *(3)*. Mother-child relationship problems are owing not only to negative interactions between a disturbed mother and a suffering newborn *(13–15)*, but also, and above all, to inadapted care practices by obstetric/pediatric teams.
2. The setting up of multidisciplinary maternity teams (obstetricians, midwives, neonatologists, psychologists, social workers, and specialists in addiction) whose

objective would be to establish a solid parent-child bond and the prevention, on the one hand, of separation and, on the other, of any consequences, owing to a chaotic family situation, on the cognitive and affective development of the child.
3. A real taking into account of the dependence on the substances consumed and the reality of the major risks to the fetus induced by brutal withdrawal (acute fetal suffering, even death *in utero*) during hospitalization for the birth or for complications. The prescription of a substitute and the medico and psychosocial support that must accompany it are well-proven methods. Withdrawal is rarely possible or durable during pregnancy but could be reenvisaged after the establishment of a solid mother-child relationship.
4. The Perinatal Network with general practitioners and specialized centers that treat these patients help to modify the negative image that these women had of the maternity wards, places that they considered as ones where they went through brutal withdrawal, were made to feel unwelcome, and where an *a priori* separation from their child was foreseen. The town-hospital perinatal network, especially with the Maternal and Child Health Centers and ambulatory child psychiatrists, allows a home-based system of support to be set up before and after birth.

All these changes in practices, of which substitution is only one element, have profoundly changed the perinatal care of these women and their children; they have achieved the goal of much warmer participation on the part of the mothers toward the welfare of their children in maternity or in neonatology, including cases of neonatal withdrawal syndrome, and have greatly reduced the level of mother-child separation.

3. RESULTS

The study includes 246 pregnant women of whom 93 (38%) followed a methadone treatment and 153 (62%) high-dose buprenorphine. The sociodemographic characteristics of the families in the two groups (Table 1) were not significantly different apart from a higher percentage of women with a partner in the high-dose buprenorphine group.

There was no difference in the age at which addiction began and the lapse of time before substitution. On the other hand, substitution was more often begun before pregnancy for high-dose buprenorphine (85%) than for methadone (71%) ($p < 0.03$). The women taking methadone were more often supervised by a specialized center (78%) than those taking high-dose buprenorphine (37%) ($p < 0.001$); the converse was true for those cared for by a general practitioner (50% under methadone and 79% under high-dose buprenorphine; $p < .001$). Sixteen percent of the women under high-dose buprenorphine used iv injection. There was no significant difference between those

Table 1
Mothers' Medicosocial Data

	Substitution by		Total ($n = 246$)	p^a
	Methadone ($n = 93[38\%]$)	High-dose buprenorphine ($n = 153[62\%]$)		
Age at this pregnancy (yr)	29.2	28.3	28.6	NS
Scolarity < primary (%)	10	19	16	NS
Foreign nationality (%)	19	25	23	NS
Income from working (%)	15	18	17	NS
Mean parity	2.3	2.0	2.1	NS
With partner (%)	49	67	61	<0.02
Own home (%)	74	81	78	NS
Health insurance (%)	98	95	96	NS
Age at beginning of addiction (yr)	18.8	20.0	19.3	NS
Delay start/substitution (yr)	9.1	7.4	8	NS
Substitution before pregnancy (%)	71	85	79	< 0.03
Supervision in specialized center (%)	78	37	53	<0.001
Supervision by general practitioner (%)	50	79	69	<0.001
HIV+ (%)	7	5	5	NS
Hepatitis C virus + (%)	73	59	64	NS

^{a}NS, nonsignificant

who were HIV seropositive and those with hepatitis C (5 and 64%, respectively, for the two groups). There was no significant difference between the two groups as far as other substances were concerned: in general, 19% for heroin, 38% for hashish, 96% for tobacco, 31% for alcohol, and 29% for benzodiazepines and/or antidepressors and/or analgesics; note that there was a higher consumption of cocaine in the methadone group (14 vs 9% in the high-dose buprenorphine group).

The figures obtained showed that there was no difference between quality of treatment during pregnancy, access to epidural analgesia, frequency of difficult births, and acute fetal distress (Table 2) in the two groups.

Women whose pregnancies were less well monitored (women in very precarious social conditions) arrived more often in the delivery room in a state

Table 2
Perinatal Data

	Methadone ($n = 93$)	High-dose buprenorphine ($n = 153$)	Total ($n = 246$)	p^a
Good prenatal care (%)	42	48	46	NS
Epidural analgesia (%)	92	85	88	NS
Emergency cesarian or forceps (%)	21	30	26	NS
Acute fetal distress (%)	26	27	26	NS
Birth weight (g) (mean)	2801	2860	2838	NS
Gestational age (wk) (mean)	38.4	38.8	38.7	NS
Premature <37wk	18	9	13	<0.04
<33wk	2.1	1.9	2.0	NS
Intrauterine growth retardation (%)	37	30	32	NS
Height <10th percentile (%)	45	34	38	NS
Head circumference <10th percentile (%)	16	9	12	NS
Apgar score at 5 min (mean)	9.9	9.8	9.8	NS
Breast feeding (%)	24	22	23	NS
Good mother-child relationship (%)	96	91	93	NS
Left with both parents (%)	51	68	62	NS
Judicial care (%)	4	3	4	NS

[a]NS, nonsignificant.

of complete dilatation of the cervix and were more often separated from their child; the level of prematurity was higher in these women than in those who were well monitored; (18 vs 9%).

Regarding the newborns (Table 2), there were no differences in neonatal mensurations, frequency of intrauterine growth retardation, APGAR scores, and percentage of breast feeding for the two groups. However, the level of prematurity was significantly higher in the methadone group (18%) than in the high-dose buprenorphine group (9%) ($p < 0.04$). There were no deaths among the children.

There was no difference in the level of breast feeding (23% overall) and the quality of the mother-child relationship, judged to be good or excellent in 93% of cases overall, between the two groups. Only 4% of the total newborns were judged to be in need of judicial care.

Table 3
Neonatal Withdrawal Syndrome Characteristics

	Methadone ($n = 93$)	High-dose buprenorphine ($n = 153$)	Total ($n = 246$)	p[a]
With Lipsitz score >0 (%)	65	65	65	NS
Mean age of beginning of neonatal withdrawal syndrome (h)	43	38.5	40	NS
Mean of maximum score	8.1	8.2	8.2	NS
Mean age of maximum score (h)	92	70	78	<0.01
Treated if neonatal withdrawal syndrome (%)	48	52	50	NS
Mean duration of treatment (d)	19	16	17	NS
Newborn transferred				
All causes (%)	32	33	33	NS
Mean hospital length of stay (d)	31	23	26	NS
Average age of regain of birth weight (d)	13	10	11	NS

[a]NS, nonsignificant.

The frequency of neonatal withdrawal syndrome (Table 3) was identical in both groups. The only significant difference was in the average age at which the maximum Lipsitz score was achieved, which was higher in the methadone group (92 h) than in the high-dose buprenorphine group (70 h) ($p < 0.01$). The percentage of children treated and the average of the maximum score were identical. A nonsignificant statistical tendency existed for the neonatal withdrawal syndrome, a little later and longer lasting under methadone than under high-dose buprenorphine. The frequency of newborn hospitalization was identical for the two groups; however, the average hospital stay was a little longer for the methadone group, but this difference was not significant and can probably be explained by a higher level of prematurity in this group. The average age for regain of birth weight was also a little later in the methadone group (13 d) than in the high-dose buprenorphine group (11 d) but was not significant.

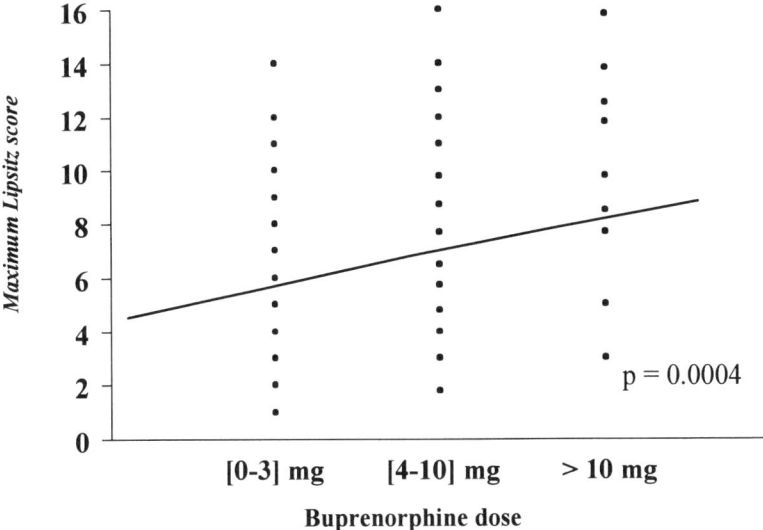

Fig. 1 Correlation between buprenorphine dose at the time of delivery and the intensity of neonatal withdrawal syndrome.

A significant correlation was found, for both groups, between the substitution treatment dose at the end of pregnancy and the intensity of the neonatal withdrawal syndrome, expressed by the maximum value of the Lipsitz score (Figs. 1 and 2). However, the dispersion, for each dose level, was such that any individual prediction of the intensity of the neonatal withdrawal syndrome, as a function of the substitution dose, is impossible.

4. Discussion

To our knowledge, this study is the first one to investigate in a comparative way (but not in a randomized double-blind one) the outcome for newborns of mothers undergoing methadone or high-dose buprenorphine substitution. Nonapproved use of buprenorphine during pregnancy in France probably explains why there was significantly more substitution begun before pregnancy with high-dose buprenorphine than with methadone. When substitution begins during pregnancy, the choice tends toward methadone but this depends on the local accessibility of a methadone program.

Women taking high-dose buprenorphine inject it in 16% of cases; this practice is worryisome when one knows the inherent risks (16). There was no significant difference between the two groups as far as associated substances

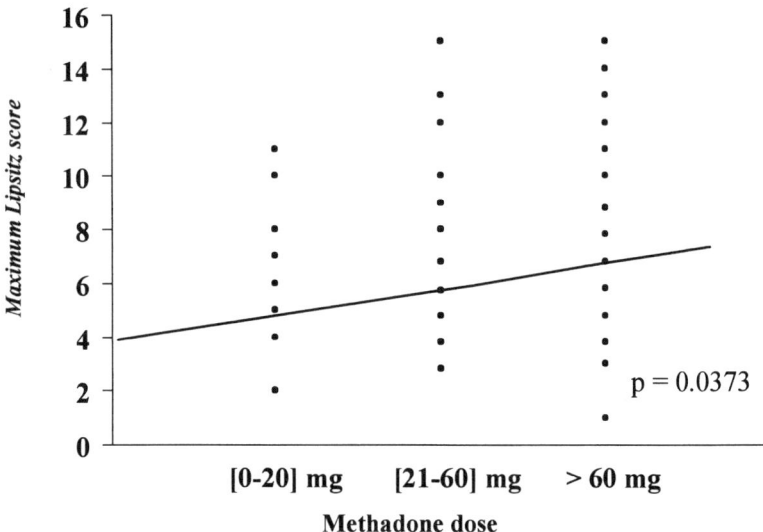

Fig. 2 Correlation between methadone dose at time of delivery and intensity of neonatal withdrawal syndrome.

are concerned; however, the information gathered was on a declarative basis, and several studies have shown that there is a wide discrepancy between what is declared and reality *(17)*.

The principal conclusion of this preliminary analysis of this cohort is that there is no major difference in perinatal prognosis between women receiving substitution treatment with either methadone or high-dose buprenorphine during pregnancy nor for their children. A finer analysis of the sociodemographic data of the two groups is under way, but there seems to be little difference between the two populations. The only differences found were: (1) a higher level of prematurity in the methadone group, but this fact will be studied more closely since it is probably owing multiple factors; and (2) the neonatal withdrawal syndrome seemed to be a bit more severe and longer lasting in the methadone group than in the high-dose buprenorphine group.

Overall, this population, cared for by a very motivated multidisciplinary group, produced data very different from those obtained from much less well cared for cohorts *(11)*; it is notable that, on comparison, there was much more supervision of the pregnancies, a decrease in perinatal pathologies, and a marked decrease in the number of infants separated from their mothers. The efforts being made at present, under the auspices of the GEGA, to generalize these practices must be pursued.

5. CONCLUSION

High-dose buprenorphine seems to be an alternative to methadone as a substitution treatment for pregnant addicts. No major difference was noted in the perinatal outcome for the two treatment groups; however, a much finer analysis of this cohort is under way.

For the a drug-dependent woman, clearly a multidisciplinary task force, in a town-hospital network, with the goal of improving the long-term prognostis for the child and his or her mother is needed.

ACKNOWLEDGMENTS

We wish to thank the following individuals for their help in collecting: E. Araujo (Versailles), H. Bastian (Paris-Bichat), M. Berthier (Poitiers), C. Boissinnot (Paris-Robert Debré), P. Bolot (Aulnay sous Bois), C. Bouderlique (Angers), J. Bouillie (Paris-St Antoine), V. Brossard (Rouen), C. Cahuzac-Lhermitte (Creil), J.X4. Chabrolle (Le Havre), F. Cneude (Lille- St Antoine), J. Dendale (Nimes), M.E. Dermer (Paris-Pitié Salpétrière), M. C. Dupard (Montreuil), M. Fiant (Mont St Aignan), C. Francoual (Paris-St Vincent de Paul), M. Gallet (Amiens), E. Bault (Paris-Les Bluets), M. Granier (Evry), B. Guillois (Caen), F. Guillot (Villeneuve St Georges), J. M. Hascoet (Strasbourg), L. Keller-Zimmerman (Mulhouse), F. Lebrun (Paris Port Royal), C. Lejeune (Colombes), H. Lucas (Saint Renan), E. Mazurier (Montpellier), P. Narcy (Saint Germain en Laye), S. Parat (Paris-Boucicault), J. M. Retbi (Saint Denis-93), M. Rolland (Toulouse), P. Sanyas (La Rochelle), J. C. Semet (Maubeuge), D. Thibault (Lille-Jeanne de Flandre).

REFERENCES

1. Kandall SR, Doberczak TM, Jantunen M, Stein J. The methadone-maintained pregnancy. Clin Perinatol 1999;26:173–83.
2. Lejeune C, Floch-Tudal C, Montamat S, et al. Prise en charge des femmes enceintes toxicomanes et de leurs enfants. Arch Pédiatr 1997; 4:263–70.
3. Randal T. Intensive prenatal care may deliver healthy babies to pregnant drug abusers. JAMA 1991;265:2773–4.
4. Jernite M, Viville B, Escande B, et al. Grossesse et buprénorphine. A propos de 24 cas. Arch Pédiatr 1999; 6:1179–85.
5. Fisher G, Etzersdorfer P, Eder H, et al. Buprenorphine maintenance in pregnant opiate addicts. Eur Addict Res 1998;4(Suppl.):32–6.
6. Fisher G, Johnson RE, Eder H, et al. Treatment of opioid-dependant pregnant women with buprenorphine. Addiction 2000;2:239–44.
7. Mazurier E, Sarda P, Boulot P. Traitement par Buprénorphine (Temgésic®) de la dépendance aux opiacés chez la femme enceinte. In: 26è Journées Nationales de la Société Française de Médecine Périnatale, livre des communications, Brest 1996.

8. Kandall SR. Treatment strategies for drug-exposed neonates. Clin Perinatol 1999;26:231–43.
9. Lipsitz PJ. A proposed narcotic withdrawal score for use with newborn infants: a pragmatic evaluation of its efficacy. Clin Pediatr 1975;14:592–4.
10. Committee on Drugs. American Academy of Pediatrics. BERLIN CM, MacCarver DG, Notterman DA, et al. Neonatal drug withdrawal. Pediatrics 1998;101:1079–88.
11. Lejeune C, Ropert JC, Montamat S, et al. Devenir médico-social de 59 nouveau-nés de mère toxicomane. J Gynecol Obstet Biol Reprod 1997;26:395:404.
12. Robins LM, Mills JL. Effect of in utero exposure to street drugs. Am J Public Health 1993;83(Suppl.):1–32.
13. Regan DO, Ehrlich SM, Finnegan LP. Infant of drug addicts: at risk for child abuse, neglect, and placement in foster care. Neurotoxicol Teratol 1987;9:315–9.
14. Davis SK. Chemical dependency in women : a description of its effects and outcome on adequate parenting. J Subst Abuse Treat 1990;7:225–32.
15. Bays J. Substance abuse and child abuse: impact of addiction on the child. Pediatr Clin North Am 1990;37:881–904.
16. Tracqui A, Kintz P, Ludes B. Buprenorphine-related deaths among drug addicts in France: a report on 20 fatalities. J Anal Toxicol 1998;22:430–4.
17. Harrison L. The validity of self-reported drug use in survey research: an overview and critique of research methods. NIDA Res Monogr 1997;167:17–36.

Index

A

Absorption, 1
Abuse liability, 16, 21, 56
Addictive power, 73
Administration, 8
Adverse effects, 60
Autopsy, 110

B

Bile concentrations, 111
Bioavailability, 1, 14
Blood analysis, 90
Breast feeding, 141

C

Ceiling effect, 22
Chemical structure, 2
Clinical trials, 31, 34
Combination with benzodiazepines, 114
Combination with CNS depressants, 111
Combination with naloxone, 18, 53
Conjugated metabolites, 95

D

Distribution, 3
Distribution in hair, 3
Doping, 97
Dose-effects, 16
Drug delivery, 71

E

Excretion, 5

F

Fatality, 110

H

Hair analysis
Health services, 70
Hepatotoxicity, 62
Heroin overdose, 74

I

Interactions with psychotropics, 20
Intravenous injection, 60, 115

M

Maintenance, 16, 122
Mass spectrometry, 92, 103
Metabolism, 5
Misuse, 74

N

Neonates' outcomes, 130

P

Pentazocine-tripelenamine, 52
Perinatal effects, 121, 140
Pharmacodynamic properties, 5
Placenta transfer, 119
Plasma concentrations, 94, 132
Pregnancy, 122, 126, 138
Prison, 76
Postmortem concentrations, 111
Procedures in prison, 77

R, S

Respiratory depression, 18, 58, 61
Safety, 21, 44
Side-effects, 44
Sublingual form, 30

T

Tablet form, 30
Therapeutic use, 70
Tissue analysis, 99
Toxicity, 19, 73
Treatment, 71, 85

U

Urine analysis, 96

W

Withdrawal symptoms, 56, 133, 142